HEALTH CARE AND THE AGED: A NURSING PERSPECTIVE

Edited by
Peter Brown
RPN, R Ger. N, DNE (Cumb.), B.A. Hons (Macq.), M.A.(Macq.), FCN(N.S.W.)
Senior Lecturer, School of Nursing
Cumberland College of Health Sciences, Sydney

WILLIAMS & WILKINS and ASSOCIATES PTY LIMITED
Sydney • Baltimore • London

National Library of Australia
Cataloguing in Publication entry

Health care and the aged.

Includes bibliographies and index.
ISBN 0 86433 023 5.

1. Geriatric nursing. 2. Aged – Care. 3. Aged – Health and hygiene.
I. Brown, Peter, 1945-

610.73'65

Typeset by Scanagraphics Pty. Limited, Sydney

Printed by Star Printery Pty. Limited, Sydney

WILLIAMS & WILKINS and ASSOCIATES PTY LIMITED
43 Herbert Street, Artarmon, NSW 2064, Australia

Contributors

Jumae Atkinson, Dip.O.Ther(LIHS,Vic), B.App.Sc.O.Ther(WAIT)
Occupational Therapist, Lower North Shore Rehabilitation and Geriatric Service, Mosman Day Care Centre, Sydney.

Laura Minasian-Batmanian, BSc, PhD(Melb)
Lecturer, Department of Biological Sciences, Cumberland College of Health Sciences, Sydney.

Pamela Brissett, RGN, DCHN, MCN(NSW)
Senior Community Nurse, Eastern Health Service, Sydney.

Peter Brown, RPN, RGerN, DNE(Cumb), BA Hons, MA(Macq), FCN(NSW)
Senior Lecturer, School of Nursing, Cumberland College of Health Sciences, Sydney.

Jean Campbell, RGN, RMN, RM'Craft, DCHN(Cumb), Grad Dip(Geront) (Cumb), FCN(NSW)
Lecturer, School of Nursing; Asst Coordinator, Associate Diploma in Community Health Nursing, Cumberland College of Health Sciences, Sydney.

Barbara Christian, RGN, RMN, RM'Craft, RPN, DNE(NSW Coll. Nursing), BA, MA(Macq), FCN(NSW)
Senior Lecturer in Nursing Science, School of Applied Science, Canberra College of Advanced Education.

Karen Heycox, BSW(UNSW)
Lecturer, Department of Social Work, University of New South Wales.

Gwen Higgins, B.Pharm(Syd), MPS, FSHP(Melb), Churchill Fellowship 1988
Pharmacist in Charge, Lidcombe Hospital, Sydney.

Sandra Longmore, RGN, RPN, RMN, DHA(Mitchell)
Director of Community Health Services, Blue Mountains Area Health Service, NSW.

Ursula Schappi, BA Hons(Macq)
Chief Ethnic Adviser, State Compensation Board, Sydney (formerly Migrant Health Education Officer, Southern Metropolitan Health Region, Sydney).

Pat Walsh, Dip OT(UK)
Occupational Therapist, Eastern Suburbs Community Rehabilitation Team, Sydney.

Preface

The growing number of older persons in the population, and the projected increase, especially of those 75 years and over, makes a greater understanding of the aged and their care increasingly important for the nurse and all other health professionals. Nursing care of the older person must play an important part in every curriculum and every nurse's attempt to keep up to date.

This book is an attempt by one nurse academic to document what he believes are some of the important aspects of gerontology which have particular relevance for the nurse caring for older adults in various community and institutional settings. Some of the information presented is oriented more to the Australian situation but overall much of the content is applicable further afield. I believe this book could be used by student nurses in the new college programs, and by nurses caring for the elderly in hospitals, nursing homes and community settings. It would also be a useful reference book for nurses' aides and other health workers involved in aged care.

I would like to express my thanks to the contributors, to my long-suffering and supportive family, and to Tracey Kellett who helped to type some of the early chapters. I am also deeply indebted to my past and present students, and to patients and clients generally who have taught me so much about old age. Finally, this book is not to be seen as an end in itself but the beginning of better things to come.

Contents

Chapter 1

Ageing and Nursing Care: An Overview

Objectives

To enable the reader to:

1. define 'ageing' and identify who the 'aged' are;
2. identify some of the myths associated with the aged which exist within society;
3. trace the reasons for the lack of interest in the aged historically and consider why there has been a renewed interest in this age group;
4. describe the universal characteristics of the aged in most societies and their demographic characteristics in Australia in particular;
5. identify the essential characteristics of a comprehensive health care system for the aged;
6. discuss some of the important issues currently facing gerontological nursing.

Who are the aged?

We use several words in our society to refer to the aged. Basically, they are known as the aged, the elderly, or older persons. If we were to consult a dictionary or thesaurus we would find that these words often carry derogatory, static or undesirable connotations.[1] The term elderly, for example, is often used synonymously with the terms ill health, disease, senility and infirmity.[2]

What is ageing then, and who are the aged? Ageing is not synonymous with illness and infirmity. It is not an event that occurs over a short period of time but a process which begins at conception and continues throughout life.[2,3] It may be seen, therefore, as an inevitable and irreversible process. While various chronological ages are used to categorise 'aged persons', 65 years and over seems to be the most widely used, although it is increasingly obvious that geriatric services more clearly relate to persons 75 years and over.[4]

This suggests that the aged might more appropriately be divided into various subgroups. Perhaps, for example, we could more correctly refer to the 'young' aged and the 'old' aged.[1,5] Still others have proposed further subdivisions.[1] Crandall[3] makes the distinction between biological age (that is, the person's physiological status and position in time relative to his potential life span), psychological age (that is, the person's ability to adapt to their environment psychologically) and social age (that is, the person's level of involvement in various roles in society). A person may not be equally old in all aspects at any one time.

Societal myths of the aged

Often old people do not feel old. Where they do, they may be reflecting society's negative attitudes and beliefs about the elderly. Undoubtedly, these attitudes and beliefs will have detrimental effects on the aged. Pallmore[6] identified 25 myths associated with the elderly. These included:

- The majority of old people are senile or demented.
- The majority of old people feel miserable most of the time.
- Most old people cannot work as effectively as younger people.
- Most old people are unhealthy and need assistance with daily activities.
- Most older people are set in their ways and unable to change.
- In general, most old people are alike.
- The majority of old people are socially isolated and lonely.

These assertions are far from the real picture one finds in daily contact with older people from all walks of life. Most old people are well and living in their own independent living situation.[1,7] Generally, most older people experience fewer work-related accidents than younger people.[8] Also, the heterogeneity of older people is perhaps greater than it has ever been.[9] Many individuals maintain physical activity and mental alertness well into their eighties and beyond, while others show changes associated with old age much earlier.[10]

Lack of interest in the aged

The existence of myths in society partly reflects a lack of knowledge of the aged generally. In the past, the aged have generated little interest.[3] To support this contention Crandall[3] notes the following:

- Because life expectancy was relatively short in the past, there was little reason to think about the aged;
- The small percentage of aged persons in society meant that they had low visibility as a group in their own right;
- Old age was not seen as a separate stage of adult development;
- During the Industrial Revolution, the aged were placed into poorhouses together with the poor, the sick, the insane and the criminal, thus denying their unique needs;
- Their concentration in small areas during urbanisation reinforced their low visibility in society;
- There existed the negative effect of stigma on the elderly;
- A high value was placed on the education of the young;
- Early psychological theorists focused on the child and child development;
- The influence of Social Darwinism emphasised the survival of the fittest;
- The interest of medicine and nursing concentrated on younger patients with acute conditions, who could be 'cured'.

To a great extent, the historical lack of interest in the elderly has been reversed,[3] although many myths still exist, perhaps for reasons other than lack of knowledge.[9]

Today more government money is being spent on the aged and their care than in any previous era.[1,8] This has been related to the fact that the elderly are more highly visible in modern society: their increased numbers, concentration in certain geographical areas, and their higher political visibility make them and their needs more apparent.[8] Then, too, the interest of behavioural scientists in the concept of stigma has generated research and interest in minority groups such as the aged.[1,9] Changes in thinking in education, medicine, nursing and behavioural science have also produced an increased interest in the elderly.[3]

Characteristics of the elderly

Acknowledging this increased interest in the aged, what do we really know about them as a group? Cowgill and Holmes (1972)[11] suggested that a small number of propositions can be stated about them which apply across most, if not all, cultures. These propositions include:

- The aged are a minority group;
- Aged females outnumber aged males, with a high proportion being widows;
- Age specific roles are ascribed to the aged which determine how they are treated by the particular society;
- As age increases, the elderly take on less physically demanding roles, but continue to serve as advisers and managers, and maintain political, judicial and civic roles.

Demographic profile

In 1976, there were 1.2 million people aged 65 years and over in Australia, making up 8.9 per cent of the total population.[12] In 1985, this figure reached 10 per cent.[13] When compared with the 610,000 aged who comprised 8.0 per cent of the population in 1947,[12] the ageing of the Australian population is evident. This trend is also seen in other Western countries.[1,3] Factors determining the proportion of aged in the population include the effects of:

- migration
- mortality
- fertility.

Traditionally, migrants have been over-representive of the workforce ages, thus decreasing the proportion of the young and the aged. The sharp decline in mortality this century was achieved mostly by declines in mortality at the younger ages, thus decreasing the proportion of aged persons. A decline in fertility (such as has been experienced in Australia) decreases the number of young people and automatically increases the proportion of workforce and aged persons.[12]

Total life expectancy has not really increased much,[1,12] although the number of people living into old age, especially those entering the group aged 75 years and over, has increased significantly.[10] In New South Wales, for example, the population aged 75 years and over will increase from 168,098 in 1978 to 284,140 in 2001.[4] More dramatic changes may be anticipated in the future with medical developments in cardiovascular and renal disease, cancer, organ transplants and Alzheimer's disease, and from research into longevity.

Development of services to meet aged needs

With the increase in the number of older people predicted for the future, it is unlikely that the wide range of needs they experience can be met by existing services. At present, those over 65 already form a large proportion of patients in medical and surgical wards in public[14] and private hospitals, and clients of community nursing services.[1,15] The number of nursing homes and the cost of beds in this sector have been highlighted in several recent government reports.[16,17] Obviously, the aged are greatly over-represented as health care consumers and thus of the health care dollar.

Acknowledging the increase in the number of aged in our society and the increased health costs involved, Mykyta[4] has proposed a single comprehensive and co-ordinated extended care service with the following components:

- assessment – domiciliary
  – hospital-based
- acute hospital care
- inpatient rehabilitation
- day care – day hospital
  – day centre
  – clubs
  – sheltered workshops
- long-stay and respite care
- accommodation – independent living
  – hostel
  – nursing home
- domiciliary care
- psychogeriatric care
- preventive programs
- education and research

Ideally, such a service would exist in every health region or subregion and would, according to Mykyta, have as its basis the following principles:

- a recognition of all influences which generate aged problems;
- a focus on the aged as a member of a social and family network, thus recognising these as a primary focus for support;
- the provision of the opportunity for the older person to stay at home and lead as normal an existence as possible;

- the recognition that the aged have the same rights of access to health care as others;
- access to health services based on multidisciplinary health assessment;
- the belief that long-term institutional care is a last option;
- institutional settings which permit as near normal a lifestyle as possible;
- the recognition that ageing does not imply illness, infirmity or senility;
- a maximal effort in the area of prevention of problems.

Ageing and gerontological nursing

Current issues in the 1980s will continue to keep the focus of nurses on the needs of the older patient or client. Regardless of the terms used – older persons, the aged, senior citizens, the elderly – attention in this textbook will focus essentially on some of the major problems facing nurses in their day-to-day contact with this subsection of the Australian population.

Historically, nursing of the aged has been viewed by many in the nursing profession in a negative light.[18,19,20,21] But gerontological nursing has emerged recently with an improved image, and Wells[22] notes the following:

- the increase in the number of textbooks, journals and other literature on gerontological nursing;
- the general interest in gerontological nursing evidenced in nursing journals;
- the increasing number of research publications in the specialty;
- higher degree opportunities in gerontology.

The number of textbooks having as their focus gerontological nursing in Australia is still somewhat limited, however. Research by Australian nurses in this area is in its infancy, and higher degree opportunities are non-existent. A substantial increase in gerontological nursing efforts is needed, especially at the tertiary education level, including a review of gerontological nursing theory and clinical opportunities in the new college-based nursing programs. Gerontological nursing textbooks, written from the Australian perspective, for both undergraduate and postgraduate students, will need to be a priority for the future.

Almost all gerontological nursing knowledge is untapped or untested in spite of the impressive and extensive clinical problems which abound; for example, incontinence, confusion, depression, constipation and falls.[13] So an equally urgent priority in the specialty is research which focuses on clinical nursing problems, that is, those problems which nurses are called upon to manage in their day-to-day contact with the older patient or client. Nurses must become more interested in these problems but must also be aware of the broader issues confronting the older patient, so that they are able to see their clinical problems in the widest context.

Summary

Ageing is a lifelong process. The aged are those over 65 years and they account for 10 per cent of the Australian population. They are a heterogeneous rather than a homogeneous group. The aged are particularly susceptible to the prejudices of society, which have their basis partly in past lack of interest in the elderly as a unique group with unique needs. Because of their increasing numbers and, therefore, influence within modern society, we are all forced to acknowledge their presence and needs. This increase in numbers requires the development of new strategies to meet health and welfare needs and costs. Gerontological nursing focuses on the clinical problems of older people. The gerontological nurse will need to develop and test new strategies of prevention and care which are based on adequate educational preparation of the nurse and tested by nursing research.

Questions

1. What is ageing?
2. Who are the aged?
3. What basis is there for dividing the aged into subgroups?
4. Identify five myths associated with the elderly.
5. Describe the available evidence which refutes the myths identified.
6. 'In the past the aged have generated little interest.' What evidence can you find to support this statement?
7. Why has there been a renewed interest in the aged?
8. Describe the almost universal characteristics of the aged in most societies.
9. Evaluate the influence of:
   (a) migration
   (b) mortality

(c) fertility

on the proportion of aged in the Australian population.

10. Outline a comprehensive health care service for the aged.
11. In what new directions does gerontological nursing need to go in Australia?

Exercise

Student-Older Person Relationship

The objectives are for the reader to:

(a) form a relationship with a healthy older person;

(b) gain insights into what it is like to grow old in Australian society.

The task is to:

(a) select an older person (not a relative) who is healthy and lives in his/her own home or in an independent living facility elsewhere in the community (for example, a retirement unit);

(b) meet at least monthly for at least one hour for a period of six months;

(c) let the older person tell their own story; state their needs; their experience of ageing; ideas about health as they were growing up and their ideas now; their thoughts about the future; their thoughts about retirement if they are about to retire;

(d) maintain confidentiality regarding privileged information;

(e) share your findings with the interviewee.

References

1. Ebersole P, Hess P. Toward healthy aging. St Louis: C.V. Mosby, 1985.
2. Syred MEJ. Changing the face of geriatric care. Nursing Times June 1981; 5-7.
3. Crandall RC. Gerontology: a behavioural science approach. Reading, Massachusetts: Addison-Wesley Publishing Co. 1980.
4. Mykyta LJ. Policy on extended care services. Sydney, Australia: Health Commission of New South Wales, 1981.
5. Murray R, Huelskoetter MM, O'Driscoll D. The nursing process in later maturity. Englewood Cliffs, New Jersey: Prentice-Hall Inc. 1980.
6. Pallmore E. Facts on aging. The Gerontologist 1977; 17(4): 315-320.
7. Job E. Eighty plus: outgrowing the myths of old age. Queensland, Australia: University of Queensland Press, 1984.
8. Howe AL, ed. Towards an older Australia. Queensland, Australia: University of Queensland Press, 1981.
9. Russell C. The aging experience. Australia: George Allen & Unwin, 1981.
10. Barrowclough F. All nurses share in the care of the old. Nursing Mirror May 1979; 13-16.
11. Cowgill DO, Holmes LD, eds. Aging and modernisation. New York: Appleton-Century-Crofts, 1972.
12. Pollard AH, Pollard GN. The demography of ageing in Australia. In Howe AL, ed. Towards an older Australia. Queensland, Australia: University of Queensland Press, 1981.
13. One in ten Australians now aged 65 or over. The Australian 12 Sept. 1985.
14. Kart CS, Metress ES, Metress JF. Aging and health: biologic and social perspectives. Menlo Park, California: Addison-Wesley Publishing Co. 1978.
15. Back B. Better ways to care for our elderly. Reader's Digest May, 1985.
16. Parliament of the Commonwealth of Australia. In a home or at home: accommodation and home care for the aged. Report from the House of Representatives Standing Committee on Expenditure. October, 1982.
17. Department of Community Services. Nursing homes and hostels review. Canberra, Australia: Australian Government Publishing Service, 1986.
18. Kayser JS, Minnigerode FA. Increasing nursing students' interest in working with aged patients. Nursing Research 1975; 24: 23-26.
19. Wilhite MJ, Johnson DM. Changes in nursing students' stereotypic attitudes toward older people. Nursing Research 1976; 25: 430-432.
20. Hart LK et al. Changing attitudes towards the aged and interest in caring for the aged. Journal of Gerontological Nursing 1976; 2: 10-16.
21. Brown P. College-based student nurses' interests in working with particular groups of patients. Journal of the Congress of Mental Health Nurses 1985; 5: 4.
22. Wells T. What does commitment to gerontological nursing really mean? Journal of Gerontological Nursing 1982; 8(8): 434-437.

Chapter 2

The Normal Ageing Process

Objectives

To enable the reader to:

1. describe the concepts and theories of ageing;
2. describe the cellular aspects of ageing;
3. describe the effects of ageing on tissues and organ systems;
4. apply this knowledge of the normal ageing process to nursing assessment and care of the elderly.

The process of ageing remains one of the mysteries of medical science. Ageing is a universal, irreversible, continuous (time-dependent) deleterious process involving growth and development that ends in death. Furthermore, it is species specific although variation between individuals does exist with respect to the degree and timing of senescent changes. The rate of ageing depends on genetic as well as environmental factors such as nutrition and stress. Homeostatic corrections in response to physiological stress are less efficient and/or slower in the aged.[1-3]

Today we are moving at an accelerating pace towards an older society. More research and improved medical care have contributed greatly to increased life expectancy in Australia. Over the decade 1971-1981 the life expectancy of Australian men and women rose by 3.45 years and 3.91 years respectively. The sex differential increased by 0.46 of a year to 7.03 years in favour of women. In Australia, females at birth now have a life expectancy of 80.72 years and males of 73.18 years,[4] the longevity of parents being reflected in the expected life duration of their offspring.[5]

However, simply adding years to life is not the answer to ageing; it must simultaneously be accompanied by an increase in the quality of life for it to be at all worthwhile. This challenge can only be overcome if the health care practitioner (in this case the nurse) has a good understanding of the normal physiologic changes associated with ageing and can thus differentiate between the changes that are due to 'normal' ageing and those related to disease processes or 'pathological' ageing. It is only then that accurate nursing assessment, prevention and care can be given to the greatly increasing numbers of the elderly.

The aim of this chapter, therefore, is to stimulate an understanding of the 'normal' ageing process.

Theories of ageing

Many different theories of ageing have been proposed simply because of the difficulty of testing them. Due to the comparatively slow rate of ageing observed in man, these theories have been based on results obtained from laboratory animal experimentation which have been extrapolated to man.[5]

Programmed Theory – this hypothesis centres around the concept that ageing is controlled by a program built into the genetic code similar to the one responsible for embryogenesis, growth and development. It further assumes that there is a 'biological clock' within the cell nucleus which monitors and sets the time within which the program is executed. Thus it may be envisaged that genes will switch on and off during growth and development according to cellular needs, but that certain 'ageing' genes exist which, when switched on, produce senescent changes which may be noticeable at both microscopic and macroscopic levels. Hence, the quality and duration of life seem to be genetically controlled and dependent on the pattern of active and inactive genes comprising this program.[6]

Error Theory – enzymes are crucial to the normal functioning cell. The greater the protein turnover rate, however, the greater the chances of accumulation of faulty proteins. In time, error-containing enzymes may therefore be produced which could in turn affect the synthesis of both structural and functional proteins. The net result would be the establishment of a positive feedback system whereby accumulation of defective proteins would affect both intra- and extra-cellular events in such a way as to lead to further faulty protein synthesis.[7,8]

Gene Redundancy – information encoded in the genes of DNA is redundant. Usually, most of the genes are repressed with only a small segment of DNA being expressed. When mutations accumulate in the active genes the redundant genes are switched on. This process continues until there is no more reserve DNA information left to draw upon and ageing occurs.[6,7]

DNA Repair Mechanisms – the rate of DNA repair is related to the life span of the species. The number of divisions that human fibroblast cells can undergo in culture has been reported to be limited to 50 divisions only, the rate of repair by DNA repair enzymes decreasing as the cells age.[7,9]

Mutation Theory – the more frequent the mitosis rate in cells, the greater the chance for age-dependent errors to creep into the genome, which are then perpetuated in transcription and translation processes. Alternatively, these mutations could arise from other sources such as radiation, chemicals and viruses. Irrespective of the causative agents, mutations may produce a totally different protein profile with a corresponding change in cell structure and function.[7,10,11]

Free Radical Theory – free radicals are short-lived molecules possessing an unpaired electron. They attack the lipids in the membranes of cells, causing significant damage through a process called lipid peroxidation. Normally, the enzyme peroxidase eliminates the presence of any free radicals in the cell by reacting with them, but with age the concentration of this enzyme decreases and hence the efficiency of this procedure drops remarkably. In old age, therefore, the body relies more heavily on the presence of antioxidants, such as vitamin E and food additives, to protect the cell from the action of any free radicals which may have formed through the action of drugs or chemicals in the environment.[6,12]

Slow Virus Infection Theory – many viruses may be found dormant in cells (without producing pathologic change) until activated by extrinsic factors (environmental or occupational) to produce such conditions as herpes simplex.[6]

Autoimmune Theory – Burnet[13] refers to the thymus as the body's 'ageing clock'. Its involution with age leads to the body switching from the use of the specific immunoglobulin G to immunoglobulin M antibody. Autoimmune diseases, cancer and general susceptibility to infections have been reported to increase with age as a consequence of increased production of autoantibodies, decreased immune surveillance and T- and B-cell mediated immunity.[6]

Stress Theory – the ability to adapt to stress is thought to depend on the genetic makeup and the nature of stress exerted on an individual. The rate of ageing is increased by such agents as radiation or continual cold.[6]

Applying this in clinical practice, we find that homeostatic corrections occur more slowly in the elderly, e.g. an elevated heart rate following exercise returns more slowly to resting levels in the old than in the young. Moreover, the efficiency of homeostatic mechanisms decreases; this failure, which is not apparent under normal conditions, becomes particularly evident under stress, e.g. accidents, change of environment, or surgery. For instance, whereas the slightest knock may cause fracture in an elderly osteoporotic bone, its young counterpart would probably require a relatively heavy fall to produce the same degree of trauma. Homeostatic errors will compound, upset the steady state equilibrium of the internal environment and ultimately lead to death.[14]

There is no one theory capable of explaining the ageing process fully. It may be that a combination of these theories as well as cellular and subcellular changes (which may in part be influenced by environmental factors) should be considered; those chosen to describe the ageing process in one individual will possibly be quite different from those chosen for another.

Cellular ageing

This section will consider the effects of ageing on a 'typical' cell (not a specific but a representative cell).

The nucleus shows altered staining characteristics and invagination of the nuclear membrane. The amount of rough endoplasmic reticulum decreases, reflecting a decreased amount of secretory protein synthesised. There is controversy in the literature about the number and size of mitochondria, the direction of change being different from tissue to tissue. Morphological changes in the mitochondria include increased fragility correlated with a decline in cellular energy supply.[15,16] The degenerating cytoplasm shows an accumulation of the pigment lipofuscin ('wear-and-tear' pigment), especially in the long-lived cells such as nerve and muscle cells. Lipofuscin concentrations can rise so high that they affect cellular function.[16,17] Sohal[18] suggested that the amount of lipofuscin is directly proportional to the degree of damage observed with ageing and that it may be related to an increase in cell destruction caused by free radicals.

The observations of the effects of age on the activities and concentrations of intracellular enzymes have been contradictory, with both increases and decreases being reported. The changes seem to be tissue specific and species and strain related. An accumulation of lipid in both blood (especially triglycerides and cholesterol) and tissues has been found in man. On the other hand, a fall in the synthesis of membrane phospholipids could explain the altered activity of the membrane-associated enzymes. The changes in cellular lipid composition, expecially those due to peroxidation and cross-linking with proteins, could account for the increased fragility of cells and organelles. Alterations in membrane receptor proteins may affect the binding and hence action of hormones.[7,9]

Effect of ageing on body systems

Integument (skin)

Epithelial tissue cells are continually replaced. The connective tissue component, particularly the dermis, hardens, loses elasticity and is responsible for the wrinkled appearance of the skin. Connective tissue contains two types of proteins: collagen, responsible for tensile strength, and elastin, responsible for elasticity. Collagen has a triple helical conformation with cross-linking between strands, while elastin has a disordered structure responsible for its rubber-like mechanical properties. Ageing is thought to involve an extra amount of cross-linking, resulting in diminished tensile strength and increased stiffness.[19]

The skin becomes pale and fragile. The epidermis, sweat glands and hair follicles atrophy and cause thinning and drying of the skin. Consequently, protection against entry of microorganisms is reduced. Together with pigmentary changes, there is an observable greying and recession of the hair of head and body, following menopause in most women and much earlier, about the thirties, in the average male. While facial hair may increase in some women, it is found to decrease in men, although eyebrows become thicker and longer. and nasal hair begins to protrude.

Nails become thick and dull as calcium is deposited, and also brittle, ridged and slow-growing.[16]

Senile pruritis may present itself as a network of minute cracks which cause discomfort and itching. Deep fissures and scaling may lead to red and weeping areas that become crusted over. Bathing should be restricted because of its drying effect on the skin. Clothes that irritate the skin should be avoided. The condition can be relieved with soothing creams. Sometimes antipruritic drugs are necessary.

Senile keratosis presents itself as a localised thickening of the skin, often in those areas of the body which have been exposed to the sun for prolonged periods of time. Senile keratoses are significant in that they can be precancerous. Initially, the lesions represent a well-demarcated red area with a few dilated blood vessels.

Seborrhoeic keratoses begin as small, demarcated, yellowish plaques. These gradually enlarge, thicken, and become darkish brown to black in colour. They become covered with a greasy, velvety-textured scale. Seborrhoeic keratoses can be removed for cosmetic reasons. For some people they can be a source of severe itching and infection.

Reduced subcutaneous fat predisposes the elderly to the development of pressure sores due to loss of padding, and reduces the skin's insulation properties. Basal metabolic rate decreases in accordance with activity and lean body mass. Homeostatic corrections are slower. All these factors contribute to a reduced capacity for thermoregulation.

Although the changes described above present no functional problems for the elderly, the nurse needs to be aware of them in order to give the best possible care.

Locomotor system

Muscles – muscle wasting as evidenced by atrophy (accumulation of lipofuscin and lipid) is reflected in a decrease in both the number and size of fibres. Hence the elderly person is weaker than his younger counterpart and, together with impaired central processing mechanisms and probable joint stiffness, he may experience:

- loss of smoothness in voluntary movement: during a movement the corrections tend to be coarse and badly adjusted, needing still further corrections, and the entire movement becomes shaky and slow;
- slower reaction time: the geriatric person may register hindrance but is incapable of taking evasive action quickly enough to prevent accidents occurring;
- less precision when attempting fine movements.[14]

These effects are less marked in elderly people who are physically active. Depending on the health status of the individual, passive or active exercise should be encouraged on a regular basis.

Bone increases in porosity and fragility, an age-related condition known as osteoporosis.[20] Women seem to be more affected than men due to the withdrawal of oestrogen following menopause which causes:

- increased osteoclastic activity with a concomitant decreased osteoblastic activity;
- decreased calcitonin secretion which upsets the delicate equilibrium normally existing between parathormone and calcitonin, so that the effects of parathormone on bone (increased calcium release) result in calcium deficient states.[16]

The hip and vertebrae are particularly susceptible to osteoporosis. Most of the elderly do not suffer ill effects from the presence of osteoporosis and, where a fracture occurs which requires internal fixation, healing takes place readily. Treatment of osteoporosis includes oestrogen replacement therapy, calcium supplements and exercise, as loss of muscle mass and inactivity seem to aggravate this condition.

Bone demineralisation caused by vitamin D deficiency is called osteomalacia and occurs particularly in the pelvis, legs and spine. Vitamin D deficiency occurs with age and causes intestinal malabsorption of calcium and hence calcium deficiency.

According to Bogduk and Twomey,[21] the shrinkage of the backbone with age with resultant diminution in height (one centimetre per decade after the age of thirty) is due to decreases in vertebral body height and not to intervertebral disc thinning as was commonly believed. Slight backache experienced in some elderly with a hunched back may possibly be due to incorrect posture and atrophy of the muscles responsible for posture and antigravity support.

Joints become drier, more fibrous (due to increased collagen and decreased elastin), less resilient and therefore stiffer. Clinically, mechanical properties and movements of joints are impaired, thus predisposing the elderly to aches and pains. Range of motion progressively decreases from adolescence and especially after the age of thirty. Complex tasks are even more difficult to accomplish by the aged if they also present with visual impairment.[14]

The nurse needs to be aware that older people cannot always support themselves while walking, standing or transferring from bed to chair, for example. It becomes important, therefore, to provide appropriate means of supporting them so as to make the most of their existing abilities and reduce the risk of injury.

Respiratory system

Atrophy and degeneration of the airway epithelial ciliary apparatus (including mucous glands) reduce the capacity for elimination of matter from the bronchial lumen. These changes render the elderly more susceptible to mechanical and infectious respiratory complications, particularly those who are sedentary, confined to bed or limited in activity. The benefits of good posture, no smoking, adequate clothing and heating as well as active and passive exercise cannot be overemphasised.

The elderly assume an abdominal type of breathing as a result of increased stiffness of the chest wall. Due to the decreased compliance of the chest wall, the abdominal type of breathing is more effective in bringing in fresh air. Calcification of the costal cartilages, osteoporosis of the thoracic vertebrae and rib cage, and degeneration (thinning) of the intervertebral discs (kyphosis) are the causes of the reduced distensibility or mobility of the rib cage. Total lung volume remains unchanged unless kyphosis or spinal problems are present (not considered part of the 'normal' ageing process), in which case lung volume and expansion capacity decreases.

The lungs, on the other hand, progressively lose their elastic recoil with age and consequently their compliance (defined as the change in volume per unit change in pressure) and functional residual capacity increases. However, since the decreased compliance of the chest wall is greater in magnitude than the increased compliance of the lung, the total compliance of the system shows an overall decrease. Breathing therefore requires more muscular effort but atrophy, with resultant weakening of respiratory muscles (intercostal, diaphragm and abdominal), limits the extent by significantly reducing the rate at which air can be moved in and out of the lungs. Vital capacity decreases while residual volume increases. The ventilatory responses to hypoxia and hypercapnia are reduced. Frequency of breathing, however, does not seem to be affected by age.

There is evidence of ventilation-perfusion mismatch with concomitant impaired arterial saturation of oxygen in the aged. Despite normal haemoglobin levels, the basal oxygen consumption decreases due to (i) loss of muscle mass, (ii) lowered 2,3, diphosphoglycerate (DPG) concentration, and (iii) a shift to the left of the oxygen dissociation curve, making it more difficult for oxygen to be released to the tissues.[14,16]

Cardiovascular system

Heart weight remains proportional to body weight. The myocardium shows signs of degeneration with lipofuscin accumulation and amyloidosis. Atrophic changes in the coronary arteries affect the blood flow and hence the availability of nutrients and disposal of wastes to and from this vital organ. With ageing, there is an increase in fibrotic tissue and loss of muscle tissue in the sinoatrial node and intranodal tracts. This causes disturbances in the heart rhythm and makes it easier for other (ectopic) centres to take over, thereby causing atrial arrhythmias.

Myocardial fibrosis will also cause stiffness of the heart chambers so that they are less able to contract and therefore respond to stress by increasing contraction strength and rate. Stroke volume and therefore cardiac output decreases, thus limiting the ability of the aged to perform physical work. The resting heart rate slows with age, the maximum heart rate being 220 minus age in years. Following exercise, however, there is an increase in heart rate and blood pressure which is more pronounced in the aged than in the young and the elevated heart rate takes longer to return to resting levels.

The stiffening of heart valves due to sclerosis and possibly calcification may cause murmurs. The nurse should suspect the possibility of heart disease whenever the elderly complain of extreme tiredness or mental confusion is apparent.

Deposition of fatty plaques in the aorta (atherosclerosis) decreases its distensibility and causes an increase in the systolic blood pressure. Thus an 80-year-old individual may have a systolic reading as high as 180 mmHg, which may be considered normal in a person of this age. This condition is referred to as senile hypertension and may precipitate thrombus formation. Since the elderly of primitive tribes or institutionalised chronic psychiatric patients do not show this kind of hypertension, environmental factors (diet and stress) have been implicated as the causative agents. Regular exercise should be included in the daily routines of the elderly to try to slow down or lower the elevated blood pressure. In those suffering from stress, relaxation techniques reinforced by biofeedback should be prescribed and adhered to on a regular basis.

Associated with the raised systolic pressure may be an increase in peripheral resistance; this in turn could elevate the diastolic pressure to 95 mmHg in the 80-year-old subject. Arteriosclerosis (hardening or loss of elasticity of the arteries) is also common in the elderly. Nor are veins spared from losing elastic tissue, so the aged are more susceptible to varicosities and hence increased venous pressure and oedema. With age also the basement membrane of capillaries becomes thicker, thus slowing down the diffusion process.[14,16,22]

The reduced responsiveness of the baroreceptor reflex to blood pressure changes leads to postural hypotension. For example, if a supine patient stands rapidly, there is an overall pressure drop due to gravity which is not compensated for by prompt arteriolar constriction. The patient thus becomes hypotensive, dizzy and feels like fainting. The nurse should be aware of the hypotensive side effects of the drug Largactil (used to calm patients) which can produce shock and death. Conditions which make orthostatic hypotension more likely, or worse, include increased body temperature or decreased blood volume due to haemorrhage, dehydration, overuse of diuretics and insufficient fluid intake. It is important to realise that hot bathing will cause dilatation of the peripheral blood vessels of the aged ('lobster look') making patients suddenly hypotensive when they stand up (vasoconstriction cannot occur quickly enough). This is why geriatric people often experience blackouts and bad falls.

Gastrointestinal system

Regeneration of the squamous epithelial cells lining the mouth is slowed and this in turn affects the healing of abrasions. Reduced salivation produces dryness in the mouth which is conducive to bacterial multiplication and hence dental caries in the aged. Gingival recession exposes more of the teeth so that they appear longer. Other changes such as missing teeth, brittle teeth and poorly functioning dentures affect ingestion and digestion functions. Atrophic changes (including neuronal atrophy) in the mucosa of the nose impair the sense of smell, and in the taste buds affect the sense of taste. (The aged have an affinity for salty or very sweet foods that require little chewing.)

Oral hygiene and care (especially in the unconscious patient) as well as normal eating habits should be encouraged in order to stimulate appetite, gastrointestinal activity, the intake of a nutritionally adequate diet and enjoyment in eating.

Atrophic changes in the gastric mucosa lead to diminished secretion of acid which may be the cause of poor food breakdown in the aged. Consequently, production of pepsinogen (needed in protein digestion) as well as mucin (essential for protection of the stomach lining from its own juices) are reduced.

Poor absorption of food in the small intestine makes it imperative for those affected to take a daily multiple vitamin to ensure at least a minimum ingestion and body utilisation of necessary vitamins and minerals.[23] Absorption may be improved and digestion promoted by eating small, spaced snacks rather than the traditional three meals a day.

Perhaps the most obvious problem associated with changes in the large intestine is constipation. In addition to decreased peristaltic activity, there is a tendency for incomplete emptying of the bowel at one time and duller nerve sensations to the lower bowel that can cause a signal for defaecation to be missed. Loss of tone affecting both internal and external anal sphincters is a major factor in faecal incontinence, which affects an increasing number of people in the later stages of ageing.

Changes in the ability to empty the gall bladder and in the physical composition of bile are the most consistent age-related changes. Statistics indicate an increase in the incidence of gallstones with age, although most cases are asymptomatic. The liver decreases in size with age but there are contradictory reports as to the changes in function. The volume of pancreatic juices is reduced. Declining appetite with resultant weight loss is related to the slowing down of bodily processes generally. Overall, the gastrointestinal system endures the test of time better than other body systems.[14,16]

Urinary system

The total percentage of fluid body weight decreases with age. Reduced nutritional intake, impaired sense of thirst, chronic illness and the use of medications may alter the fluid volume and composition. This could lead to impaired cardiac, renal and mental function. Therefore, although the senescent kidney is able to maintain adequate function to cope with a lower metabolism, the adaptive mechanisms responsible for maintaining constancy of volume and composition of extracellular fluid are impaired. This is especially evident under conditions of stress, such as acute illness (which may delay recovery and prolong hospitalisation).

Structural as well as vascular changes contribute to declining renal efficiency. Atrophic changes in the kidney include (i) loss of renal mass due to a reduction in the number of nephrons, (ii) thickening of the basement membrane of the Bowman's capsule, (iii) degenerative changes in the tubules and (iv) variable sclerotic changes in the walls of renal vessels. Consequently, glomerular filtration rate, the secretion and reabsorptive capabilities of the renal tubules, and renal plasma flow all decrease. Thus, the ability of the kidney to concentrate or dilute urine and regulate acid-base balance is reduced.[14]

The ureters, urethra and bladder become less elastic and so the tone of these structures is decreased. In the bladder, these changes could impair its complete emptying (larger residual volume) due to degeneration, lessened reflexes and bad posture. Bladder capacity declines[20] and the signal to urinate does not occur until capacity is reached. This situation leads to frequency and urgency. Nocturia is common in the elderly. Approximately two-thirds of the aged population wake two or more times a night to urinate.[24] These conditions are often annoying to the older person.

The bladder outlet in older women exhibits a high incidence of funnelling which is probably the result of deterioration of the pelvic diaphragm. If the latter is weak it can contribute to imperfect closure of the bladder outlet, causing leakage and stress incontinence. Stress incontinence occurs when there is a sudden rise in intravesical pressure such as occurs in coughing or sneezing.[24]

Enlargement of the prostate with age is the most common cause of bladder dysfunction in males. The uninhibited neurogenic bladder is probably the most important factor leading to incontinence. Although there may be no escape from incontinence or bladder weakness for the very old, it should not be allowed to become degrading. The aged person should be encouraged to adopt the aids available for both day and night incontinence to minimise the work of those looking after them and to improve their self-esteem.[25]

Generally, good voiding habits and regular fluid intake should be encouraged and older people should be taught the role of fluids in keeping the urine free from bacteria. When an aged person is hospitalised, the nurse will often be responsible for ascertaining that the daily intake of fluids and output is adequate.

Endocrine system

The levels of hormones in the circulation are determined by the concentrations of specific receptors and the relative rates of synthesis and secretion versus degradation of these hormones. Homeostatic mechanisms come into play to ensure that the correct concentrations of individual hormones are maintained and thus the internal environment does not deviate from steady state. Endocrine failure does not appear to be part of the 'normal' ageing process. Diminishing reserves rather than endocrine failure seems to be the reason for any deficiencies observed, especially in situations of stress.[14]

Susceptibility of individuals to diabetes mellitus increases with age, particularly in the obese elderly, who show a decrease in glucose tolerance. Whether this is due to a decreased number of receptors and hence reduced insulin sensitivity, or to diminished pancreatic B-cell secretion in response to hyperglycaemia, is not yet established. Receptor loss, however, seems to be the cause of most endocrine deficiencies so this may possibly explain the reason for the increased incidence of type II (maturity-onset) diabetes.

Pituitary function remains within normal limits (except for lower serum prolactin levels in women after menopause). Thyroid activity and basal metabolic rate both decrease with age. Postmenopausal women show an occurrence of osteoporosis due to increased parathormone secretion by the parathyroid gland. The degradation of this hormone slows with age so that the elevated circulating levels are maintained, unlike the case in men. Plasma glucocorticoid levels remain unchanged, but the decreasing renin levels with age lead to a concomitant fall in the aldosterone concentration. These changes, together with those in antidiuretic hormone secretion, may give rise to decreased blood pressure, tissue turgor and orthostatic hypotension.[14,16,26]

Central nervous system: special senses

Eye – takes on a sunken appearance as orbital fat decreases with age. Consequently, there is a reduction in the field of vision of the elderly, especially if ptosis (drooping eyelids) is also present. Degeneration of the retina, particularly the macula, causes poor sight to occur gradually. Visual acuity (sharpness of vision) and tolerance of glare decreases as receptors of the fovea are lost. Presbyopia is a common condition encountered in the elderly, characterised by an inability to focus on things close at hand. With age, the lens loses elasticity, it cannot change shape easily and hence its ability to accommodate becomes increasingly limited. The rate at which accommodation occurs is also slowed because of the deterioration in ciliary muscle performance.[27]

Other age-related changes include increased intraocular pressure, contracted pupils, impaired colour vision (the aqueous humour becomes pigmented and so blue, green and violet are progressively harder to perceive clearly), slowing of adaptation to the dark, drying of the cornea, decreased lacrimation and muscae volitantes (specks seen floating in front of the eyes).[14,16]

Adequate lighting and appropriate spectacles can result in a significant improvement in behaviour stemming from sensory deprivation.

Ear – shows a progressive perceptive hearing loss occurring with age (presbycusis). This is due to:

- loss of elasticity in the basilar, Reisner's and tympanic membranes;
- loss of hair cells from the organ of Corti and semicircular canals (contributing to loss of balance and posture);
- loss of neurones from temporal cortex;
- atrophy of striae vascularis;
- increased wax accumulation; and
- decreased vibration of the auditory ossicles.

These changes cause the elderly to lose the ability to hear higher frequencies. In the early stages, this may not cause problems in normal conversation but as the condition progresses communication may be affected. Speech can be heard but words cannot be discriminated (cortical impairment), especially against background noise. Loss of sound orientation is also common in the elderly,[14,16] so noise reduction and appropriate pacing of conversation should always be practised when talking to an aged person in order to improve communication. Problems with hearing can be devastating and can lead to isolation of the elderly; they should therefore be encouraged to wear hearing aids.

Central nervous system: brain and spinal cord

Brain loses bulk with atrophy of the cerebral gyri and widening and deepening of the sulci. These changes are not incompatible with normal intellectual function, as the brain possesses a tremendous reserve capacity. Most of the elderly are able to function adequately unless rushed or confronted with a new environment or routine. However, mental agility slows down and forgetfulness becomes progressively evident (mainly short-term memory is affected); this makes learning increasingly more difficult with advancing years. The elderly become more and more preoccupied with their own thoughts and the past and less interested in what is going on around them, such as the activities of family or society.[28-30]

The central processing mechanisms are impaired because of loss of neurones and a fall in the number of synaptic connections due to axonal and dendritic degenerations. The reduction in the concentration of synaptic neurotransmitters which occurs with ageing further interferes with central processing. Atrophy of cells in the cerebellum causes a decrease in muscle tone and muscle co-ordination with age. The spinal cord also suffers from cell loss and different parts of the brain and spinal cord may age at different rates. As a consequence, tendon reflexes are impaired and the posterior column processes deteriorate.[31]

Cerebral blood flow and oxygen consumption rate decrease. Degenerative changes observed in the neurones include lipofuscin accumulation, cytoplasmic RNA, mitochondria and enzyme loss, and senile plaques and neurofibrillary tangles (predisposing to senile dementia).[14,16,32]

Sensitivity to pain, touch, heat, cold and joint position may be abnormal. The nurse needs to be aware that the older person's response to pain may produce a different clinical picture to the traditional one. For example, the retrosternal crushing pain associated with a myocardial infarction may be completely missing. The nurse, therefore, must be alert to other features which will indicate the presence of a serious illness. Changes in the normal pain signals have implications too for the creation of pressure areas and tissue damage caused by heat or cold.

Genital system

In the female over forty, ovarian failure leads to loss of the reproductive function, this being characterised by the climacteric (the time taken for the menstrual cycle to become irregular and stop). This period may be anything from a few months to several years. As a result, some women may experience hot flushes, irritability, sweating, fatigue, depression, anxiety and osteoporosis. Although oestrogen therapy can overcome these symptoms, they will linger for a longer period of time. The male reproductive system, on the other hand, continues to produce male sex hormones well into old age although production gradually declines. The decrease affects muscle strength and the number of viable sperm produced.

The ovaries, uterus, fallopian tubes, cervix, vagina, vulva and mammary glands (alveoli and ducts are lost) show different extents of atrophy in postmenopausal women. The uterus becomes more fibrous. The vulva and vaginal walls thin, secretion is reduced and in the vaginal pH rises, resulting in changes of the flora. Hence the vulva and vaginal walls become more susceptible to injury and infection. The breasts droop (due to the loss of adipose tissue) and the nipples become smaller and less able to become erect. Pubic hair only becomes scarce in the latter years of life.

In the male, the testes become more fibrous and the seminiferous tubules thicken. The germinal epithelium degenerates, reducing sperm production. The prostate gland enlarges. The penis maintains its ability to become erect although more physical stimulation may be necessary to achieve an erection. Ejaculations are slower and less forceful.[16,33]

Summary

Although the elderly function quite well under normal conditions, compensatory homeostatic mechanisms become less efficient and/or too slow under stressful situations (e.g. haemorrhage, dehydration, electrolyte imbalance). A reduction in the reserve capacity, and an inability to rely on the functioning of certain vital organs, which are an integral part of the homeostatic mechanism, may be the reason for the upset in steady state which leads to failure and eventual death.

Questions

1. Describe the mutation theory as one of the pathophysiologic mechanisms in senescence.
2. Metabolism slows down in the elderly. What are the possible reasons for this?

3. What criteria do you envisage a 'youth serum' should have in order to slow down the ageing process?
4. Describe the cardiovascular causes underlying the blackouts and bad falls that geriatric people often experience.
5. The elderly often complain of loss of sensitivity to high frequency tones. Describe two degenerations of the ear that may cause this.
6. (a) What do you understand by the term climacteric?
   (b) State five symptoms associated with this condition.
7. Name a predisposing factor causing impairment of bladder control, leading to incontinence in the elderly.
8. Explain why fibre is especially important in the diet of the elderly.
9. Describe two effects of ageing on the skin.

Puzzle

Unlike normal cells, cancer cells do not seem to age and die. Explain this phenomenon by using your knowledge of the mechanisms of ageing and the references cited below.

References

1. Comfort A. The biology of senescence. New York: Elsevier, 1979.
2. Lamb MJ. Biology of aging. New York: John Wiley and Sons, 1977.
3. Finch C, Hayflick L. Handbook of the biology of aging. New York: Van Nostrand Reinhold, 1977.
4. Australian Bureau of Statistics 1986 Census.

5. Everitt AV, Burgess JA. Hypothalamus, pituitary and aging. USA: Charles C. Thomas, 1976.
6. Groer ME, Shekleton ME. Basic pathophysiology, C.V. Mosby, 1979.
7. Davies I. Ageing. Edward Arnold Ltd, 1983.
8. Brocklehurst JC. Textbook of geriatric medicine and gerontology. New York: Churchill Livingstone, 1978.
9. Behnke JA, Finch CE, Moment GB. The biology of aging. New York: Plenum Press, 1978.
10. Kohn RR. Principles of mammalian aging. New Jersey: Prentice-Hall, 1971.
11. Rockstein M. Theoretical aspects of aging. New York: Academic Press, 1974.
12. Strehler BL. Time, cells and aging. New York: Academic Press, 1962.
13. Burnet FM. An immunological approach to aging. Lancet 1970; 2: 358.
14. Adams GF. Essentials of geriatric medicine. New York: Oxford University Press, 1981.
15. Miquel J, Economos AC, Fleming J, Johnson JE, Jr. Mitochondrial role in cell aging. Experimental Gerontology 1980; 15: 575.
16. Kenney RA. Physiology of aging. Chicago, London: Year Book Medical Publishers Inc. 1982.
17. Viidik A. Lectures on gerontology. Academic Press IA, 1982.
18. Sohal RS. Age pigments. New York: Elsevier/North-Holland Biomedical Press, 1981.
19. Hall DA. Aging of connective tissue. London: Academic Press, 1976.
20. Eliopoulos C. Health assessment of the older adult. Menlo Park, California: Addison-Wesley Publishing Co. 1984.
21. Bogduk N, Twomey LT. Clinical anatomy of the lumbar spine. Churchill Livingstone, 1987.
22. Goldman and Rockstein. Physiology and pathology of aging. Academic Press, 1975.
23. Ebersole P, Hess P. Toward healthy aging. St Louis: C.V. Mosby, 1981.
24. Kart GS, Metress ES, Metress JF. Aging and health: biologic and social perspectives. Menlo Park, California: Addison-Wesley Publishing Co. 1978.
25. Yeates WK. Normal and abnormal bladder function. In Willington FL ed. Incontinence in the elderly. London: Academic Press, 1976.
26. Gusseck DJ. Endocrine mechanisms and aging. Adv in Gerontol Res 1974; 4: 105.
27. Fisher RF. Presbyopia and the changes with age in the human crystalline lens. J Physiol 1973; 228: 165.
28. Botwinick J, Storandt M. Memory, related functions and age. C.C. Thomas, 1974.
29. Butler R, Lewis M. Aging and mental health. St Louis: C.V. Mosby, 1982.
30. Allison RS. Mental impairment in the aged. Philadelphia: M. Jacobs, 1964.
31. Gershon S, Terry R. Neurobiology of aging. New York: Raven Press, 1976.
32. Adams GF. Cerebrovascular disability and the aging brain. London: Churchill Livingstone, 1974.
33. Timiras PS, Vernadakis A. Hormones in development and aging. MTP Press, 1982.

Chapter 3

Preventive Care in Old Age

Objectives

To enable the reader to:

1. recognise the importance of preventive health care in old age, in particular the need for the older person to pay attention to nutritional and dietary needs, exercise and keeping active mentally;
2. recognise the importance of good nutrition for older people and identify their dietary needs;
3. discuss some of the reasons for poor nutrition in old age;
4. describe the effects of poor nutrition on the older person;
5. identify special problems (including those experienced by the older migrant) related to diet in old age and the dietary modifications which may be necessary;
6. discuss the role of the nurse in relation to nutrition and diet in the care of the aged;
7. discuss the benefits of physical and mental activity in old age;
8. describe active and passive exercises suitable for the elderly;
9. identify why many of the aged do not participate in physical activities or keep mentally active;
10. recognise how physical and mental activity may be promoted in old age;
11. evaluate the older person's ability to learn new material and benefit from education.

Older adults are continually reminded of their health. They may, for example, experience increasing stiffness of joints or decreasing energy reserves. Preventive health care, although not able to halt the advance of the ageing process, can reduce the effects of existing problems and prevent further complications and dependency.[1]

For the most part, the elderly are healthy and this should be encouraged. For those with chronic illness or disabling conditions, health maintenance and promotion should be directed towards keeping them healthy in their day-to-day functioning.[2] Paying attention to nutritional and dietary needs, exercise and keeping mentally active, will help to keep the elderly generally healthy, and those who have chronic and disabling conditions well.[3,4] Even in chronic illness it is possible to achieve and maintain an optimal level of wellness.[4] To achieve or maintain wellness, one needs to give attention to several areas of functioning. This chapter will discuss nutritional and dietary awareness, physical fitness and keeping mentally active.

Nutritional and dietary awareness

Food is essential for the maintenance of biological life and psychosocial well-being.[4-7] The older person's nutritional status will be influenced by many factors, including:

- the body's unique utilisation of the food that is eaten;
- personal health and well-being;
- income, lifestyle, housing, geographic location;
- availability of services to meet physical, social, and emotional needs.[4,8,9]

Diet and longevity

Surveys of the long-lived populations of the world (in Peru, Pakistan and Russia) have indicated that one of the factors involved in longevity is diet.[9] The daily per capita intake of the three communities studied ranged from 1200-1900 calories. The villages observed in Peru and Pakistan were agricultural communities, and the populations ate a largely vegetarian diet. The village in the Caucasus (Russia) was a mixed agricultural and dairy economy. Unfortunately, no conclusive results were identified.

Specific mechanisms or nutrients responsible for the ageing process are yet to be found, but there seems little doubt that nutrition is one of the most significant environmental factors in resistance to disease.[4,7,8,10,11] Diet contributes significantly to many degenerative diseases affecting elderly people in Western society[5,12] (see the section below on special diet-related problems in old age).

Social aspect of food

Food plays an important role in society and the preparation and consumption of food are seen as social events.[5] Its preparation, for example, gives pleasure to many and also provides them with important roles. Eating can also be pleasurable in terms of the taste, texture and odours of the food being eaten. Unfortunately, the social importance of food declines with increasing age.[10] Preparation of food may become more difficult because of physical limitations. Financial difficulties may severely limit the types of food that can be bought. Loss of teeth and normal ageing changes, such as impaired sense of smell and touch, may make foods seem tasteless. The social aspects of food may be lost when a spouse dies or is hospitalised.[4,5,9,10,12,14]

Nutritional needs of the elderly

The aged experience many of the nutritional problems of other age groups,[10,12,15] but they also have a greater probability of nutritional problems because of an increasing incidence of disease, which creates a physiological disruption in the digestive process.[7,12,14]

People in the older age group generally require the same amount of protein, vitamins and minerals as they did when they were younger, but energy needs are usually reduced.[13] This is due to a reduction in physical activity, as well as reduced requirements to maintain body functions.[9,12] As we shall see later, if the joule value of the older person's diet is not reduced, an overweight problem is likely to occur.[4,5,14]

Current evidence seems to suggest that requirements for nutrients do not decrease with age.[9] Good nutrition in old age means that all the essential nutrients (carbohydrates, fat, protein, vitamins, minerals and water) are adequately supplied and utilised to maintain health and a sense of well-being. There are various books available that give detailed accounts of these nutrients. Some examples of nutritional requirements for the older adult are given in Table 3.1.

Dietary fibre and water are also very important dietary essentials. Water is important for proper elimination and fluid balance. Many older people have problems associated with constipation and dehydration and it is essential that elderly people drink at least six or seven glasses of water a day. Fibre facilitates the absorption of water, increases bulk and improves

Table 3.1 Special Nutritional Considerations for the Older Adult

Nutrient	**Comments**
Protein	1g/kg body weight; ¼-½ should be of animal source, the remainder of plant origin; sources of protein are meat, fish, poultry, eggs, cheese, dry beans, peas and nuts.
Fat	The body's need for fat remains relatively unchanged with age; fat should make up 20% of total caloric consumption; polyunsaturated fats of plant origin should be emphasised.
Iron	Adequate intake of iron is necessary to prevent iron deficiency problems; iron may be obtained from beans, cereals, wholegrain breads.
Potassium	Potassium deficiency is generally associated with diuretic therapy, renal disease and diarrhoea; the main sources of potassium are citrus fruits and milk.
Vitamin C (ascorbic acid)	A frequently reported deficiency in the elderly; deficiency may be related to the cost of foods rich in vitamin C; sources include oranges, lemons, tomatoes, leafy greens and potatoes.
Vitamin A	Intake may be inadequate as the older person finds that vegetables containing vitamin A are hard to chew and digest; sources include green vegetables, carrots, sweet potato, watermelon and liver.
Vitamin B_1 (thiamine)	Deficiency may result in loss of appetite, indigestion, fatigue, neuritis, irritability; sources include pork, beef, liver, legumes and whole grains.
Vitamin B_2 (riboflavin)	Deficiency may result in dermatitis, eye irritation; sources include milk, liver, enriched cereals.
Vitamin B_6 (pyridoxine)	Deficiency may result in anaemia; sources include wheat, corn, meat, liver.
Vitamin B_{12} (cobalamin)	Absorption of vitamin B_{12} seems to decrease with age; liver, milk, eggs and green vegetables are excellent sources.
Niacin	Deficiency may cause neuritis, dermatitis, lassitude, weakness.
Folic acid	Deficiency may result in megaloblastic anaemia and dementia; sources include green leafy vegetables, beans and peas, wholegrain bread, cereals and liver.

intestinal motility.[4,7,10] Bran or wholegrain breads and cereals will greatly enhance the older person's dietary fibre intake.

Studies have shown that a 5 per cent reduction in calorie needs per decade occurs from age 55-75, and the rate of reduction increases to 7 per cent per decade after age seventy-five.[12] A diet of 1650-2200 calories would seem to be appropriate for the older person,[7,12] but this reduced need for calories is often not reflected in the diets of older people. For example, poor protein intake in the elderly is often caused by the high cost of protein-rich foods, poor chewing ability, malabsorption problems and poor education about what an adequate diet in old age should comprise. It is not surprising that cheaper carbohydrate foods are substituted which have a higher caloric value.

Special diet-related problems in old age

Obesity

The relationship between obesity and degenerative disease is strong enough to suggest that weight reduction should be a means of preparing for old age. A tendency towards obesity may be the result of genetic inheritance, or eating patterns, or may have its genesis in losses experienced over the life span.[4,5,12] A recent study in Sydney found that 47 per cent of the older persons studied considered themselves overweight.[16]

Being old and overweight can cause several problems. For those with arthritis, excessive weight can further decrease mobility. It can cause the older individual to experience fatigue on minimal effort and will generally reduce life satisfaction and longevity. Increased weight will make the older person more prone to falls. Other health-related problems associated with obesity include arteriosclerosis, cardiovascular disease, hypertension, respiratory difficulties and diabetes mellitus. Where it occurs in the older age group, the onset of Type II diabetes appears directly related to the degree of obesity experienced.[4,5,8,12]

Here the dietary modifications should be closely monitored and reviewed by the health team and the diet fully explained to the sufferer. For those who are borderline diabetics, dietary needs should be closely monitored by the patient's doctor, dietitian and nurse. An awareness and recognition of the emotional and behavioural factors that may be present is indispensible in helping the older person to come to grips with the problem and to want to lose weight.

Dehydration

The aged are vulnerable to fluid and accompanying electrolyte imbalances. Institutionalised patients are particularly prone to dehydration, especially those who are unable to obtain fluids for themselves. Generally, infections and hot weather will deplete the older individual of much needed body fluids.[4,7] Adequate fluid intake is considered to be 1½-2 litres daily.[12] Those who are unable to take fluids for themselves must be assisted to do so. Water should be readily accessible, especially to those who are bed- and chair-fast.[4,7,8]

Malnutrition

A problem for many aged persons is that of malnutrition. Those at risk include people with severe psychosocial problems or eating problems related to mechanical difficulties. Specific problems include low income, social isolation and loneliness, alcohol abuse, confusion, loss of dentures, ill-fitting dentures, inability to feed oneself, and neurological defects.[5-9] Malnutrition can make older individuals confused, tired and more prone to accidents.[12]

Barriers to good nutrition in old age

There are many good reasons why an older person's appetite may be poor. An impaired sense of smell and taste, for example, may lead to a reduction in appetite arousal, and so to a poorer digestive response. Chewing is less effective because of weaker facial muscles and problems with existing teeth and dentition.[13] Diminished efficiency of the digestive system is reflected in reduced secretion of digestive juices and enzymes. Some of the food passing through the digestive system will not be metabolised, making it unavailable for the body's use. As there is a close relationship between digestion and one's emotional state, anger or fear may spoil the appetite or lead to feelings of nausea and indigestion.

Elderly people living alone may feel that preparation of meals is too much trouble, or they may not be able to afford adequate nutrients. As physical and cognitive changes occur in old age, the task of food preparation may become increasingly difficult. For example, failing eyesight and tremulous hands or loss of strength can make the operation of stoves and electrical appliances dangerous and the use of knives and forks more difficult. Older people living alone may have little incentive to cook for themselves.

Fixed incomes which do not keep pace with inflation will limit what nutrients the older person can buy. Many become poor after retirement and find it difficult to change their lifestyles. Others have had an inadequate formal education and limited life experiences and do not always understand their nutritional needs in old age or how to manage available finances. Still others live in inadequate accommodation which does not allow for the proper preparation and storage of food.[4,6-8,10,11,14] Kendig[17] found that a considerable number of older people, who were private boarders, lodgers and renters, were unable to prepare their own meals.

Special diets entail additional costs, shopping and preparation. Transportation to and within shopping centres may be difficult or absent. Certain specific conditions also have important effects on the nutritional status of the elderly. These include:

- depression
- physical disability
- malabsorption and gastrointestinal disorders and discomfort

- mental deterioration
- inadequate knowledge of dietary principles
- bereavement
- removal from usual cultural patterns
- sensory defects
- intentional starvation[4,7,15,18].

Changing longstanding dietary habits will be difficult and in some instances almost impossible. Disturbance of lifelong habits, for example, can often result in stress, anger, depression and other regressive behaviours.

Nursing roles in relation to nutritional needs of the aged

Nurses must practise under the assumption that nutrition and health are intrinsically related, so it follows that promotion of good nutrition in the elderly becomes an important nursing role. The nurse can determine the nutritional status of the aged patient by:

- physical assessment;
- comprehensive evaluation of food consumption and activity;
- taking a medical history;
- measuring height, weight, fat, and muscle mass;
- compiling relevant laboratory data as they relate to suspected nutritional deficiencies.[4,8,11]

Assessing food consumption

To help evaluate a person's nutritional status, a comprehensive evaluation of food consumption should be made. The patient can be encouraged to keep an account of the kinds and amounts of food and liquids ingested over a one week period.[11] It would not be difficult for the nurse to construct a relevant chart for this purpose. The data obtained can then be compared with the recommended daily allowances for a person of that height and age. Additional information for assessment purposes will include:

- food likes and dislikes
- difficulties with chewing
- food purchasing behaviour
- food storage and preparation
- budgeting behaviour
- activity and exercise levels
- special dietary considerations.

The nurse also needs to be aware of the existence of such community resources as Meals-on-Wheels,[19,20] weight reduction programs, migrant services and dietitians' services.

Client involvement

Obviously, any nutritional changes to be effected will be brought about only by the direct involvement of the patient/client. The patient has to know why dietary changes need to be made and what those changes are. The desired outcomes need to be made explicit. Radical dietary changes will not usually be called for as these would be too difficult for some of the reasons identified earlier. Often modifications of the older person's lifestyle and dietary habits will suffice. It is important to develop a plan of action that is oriented to the individual older person's particular situation. The client may need suggestions for making balanced, easy-to-fix meals or advice on how to control weight gain through caloric restriction and sensible exercise.

Weight loss based upon emotional factors or apathy may be overcome by giving the older person smaller, more frequent meals and supplementary feeds if hospitalised. For the patient with weakened facial muscles and problems with dentition, food should be of a kind that does not require extensive mastication.

When encouraging an older person to try new foods or make other changes in dietary habits, remember that a strong set of food likes and dislikes has been developed over many years. Any changes, therefore, should be attempted gradually. Offer plenty of encouragement. If the older person is very resistant to change, accept this in order to maintain rapport.[4,7,8,10,14]

Five food group plan

An easy set of guidelines for planning nutritious meals is the five food group plan.[4,13] This will provide all the older person's nutritional needs if the recommended amounts from each of the groups are consumed daily. The plan can form a basis for preparing the shopping list and selecting the most appropriate foods from the supermarket. The five food groups are:

- bread and cereals
- fruit and vegetables
- meat, poultry, fish
- milk and cheese
- butter, fats and oils

There is usually no need to take vitamin supplements unless there are demonstrable deficiencies.[12] If digestion or absorption of food is poor, or the diet poorly chosen, a multi-vitamin may be helpful.[5] Lowered levels of folate and vitamin C have been found in long-term residents in institutions, so the need to supplement these nutrients should not be overlooked.[21] Salt and salty foods should be used in moderation.

The nurse should be aware that there are many ways for the elderly to minimise food costs without losing out on nutritional value. Good planning is the starting point and further suggestions appear in Table 3.2.

Table 3.2 Helpful Hints to Reduce Food Costs

- Plan menus ahead.
- Make out a shopping list.
- Avoid impulsive buying.
- Shop only once or twice weekly.
- Be familiar with the price of foods.
- Buy fruit and vegetables in season.
- Freeze bread to keep fresh.
- Make good use of leftovers.
- Store food correctly.
- Keep food well covered and refrigerated.

Relatives may be able to help in practical ways by providing a small refrigerator, easy-to-use stove or microwave oven for the older person's use. Relatives and neighbours may also be asked to include additional food items in their own shopping for older people who are unable, for various reasons, to get out to do their own shopping. Eating a meal occasionally with the older person may help them to maintain an interest in eating.

Community services

Alternatively, or in addition, help may be sought from the local Meals-on-Wheels organisation. This community-based service is funded by the Commonwealth Government Department of Social Security, which provides a subsidy of 50 cents for each meal served and an extra five cents if a vitamin C supplement, such as orange juice, is provided to the older client. Few of the non-English speaking migrant aged use Meals-on-Wheels, partly because most services have provided only Australian style food until recently. In 1983 the New South Wales Meals-on-Wheels Committee suggested a distribution plan[22] whereby 'ethnic' foods could be provided through hospital and Meals-on-Wheels kitchens. It is anticipated that in the near future Greek and Italian dishes will be served in the inner-western Sydney area, with a view to expanding the variety of foods to be served to other migrant communities throughout the metropolitan area. It will be important for migrant community members to be involved in delivering the meals.

The nurse can be instrumental in bringing together older people for meals, and in locating centres for senior citizens that serve hot meals at low cost.

Education programs in nutrition must be geared to where the older people live and deal with the particular problems that they experience. The nurse must, for example, consider their social, economic, cultural and educational circumstances. Current physical and mental health problems will also be important considerations.[4,8] There is a real need for printed materials on nutrition that are suitable for older people of different levels of income and education. This material should be relevant and practical. Direct contact will always be important though as printed materials are often thrown away.

Physical activity

Physical activity can have many positive effects on the older person. Johnson-Pawlson and Koshes,[23] for example, argue that it will increase the ability to be physically active, help to minimise the number and severity of acute problems, reduce disability associated with acute or chronic illness and, in general, maintain a sense of well-being. Moreover, it has been found that when older subjects participated in a regular monthly activity program, their self-esteem score increased and depression scores decreased significantly.[24]

Bassett, McClamrock and Schmelzer[25] sought to determine whether exercise would improve the flexibility, quadriceps strength and balance of elderly men and women as a result of a 10-week, non-strenuous, progressive exercise program. Many participants said that they felt better and could get around more easily after joining the program, and shoulder, hip and knee flexibility were found to have increased significantly. Also, strong group cohesiveness formed and continued after the course.

Twenty-three geriatric patients from a mental institution were studied to determine their response to a 12-week program of physical activity.[26] Results indicated that daily activity level increased, patient self-care was upgraded, and activity tolerance levels increased.

De Vries' studies[27] of physical activity in old age indicated that programs improved heart muscle tone, decreased blood pressure and body fat, and improved respiration. Goldberg and Fitzpatrick[28] found that movement therapy increased the morale and self-esteem of the older people who took part in their study.

Benefits of physical activity

The benefits of physical activity in terms of quality and quantity of life seem to be evident from a review of some of the studies available. It is probable, though, that the aged who are currently physically active have been that way all their life and continue into old age to have the most positive attitude towards exercise and activity. This indicates that the benefits of exercise and physical activity generally should be promoted early in life.[10,16]

Traditionally, physical activity has been regarded as an occupation of younger age groups.[5] Indeed, Banks[6] suggests that many view the aged as sedentary beings. But it is through activity that many physical, psychological and social benefits may be gained.[7] Physical activity aids respiration and the circulatory, digestive, excretory and musculoskeletal functions. It also has significant effects on mental health in that those who are active feel better in and about themselves. Activity will often bring the older adult into contact with others, and will also help to reduce the effects of chronic health problems.[7]

Active and passive exercise

Starting unaccustomed physical activity the day after retirement is a good way of doing oneself an injury.[29] Obviously, before starting, a thorough physical check-up will be necessary. A positive attitude towards exercise and regular practice should be established as early as possible.[10] Physical activity may be active or passive. Table 3.3 identifies a range of active exercises. A range of passive exercises are also possible (see Table 3.4).

Table 3.3 Active Exercises suitable for the Elderly

- Bicycling
- Calisthenics
- Jogging
- Weight lifting
- Swimming
- Walking
- Dancing
- Golf
- Ping-pong
- Outdoor and indoor bowls
- Lawn mowing and gardening
- Tennis
- Walking to the shops
- Walking a pet
- Washing the car

Table 3.4 Passive Exercises suitable for the Elderly

• Knitting, tapestry, crochet	• Flexion and extension exercises
• Exercises during a shower or bath	• Dishwashing, as a means of exercising stiff finger joints
• Deep breathing and limb exercises	• Foot, leg, shoulder and arm exercises while watching TV
• Maintaining pets	• Stretching exercises
• Passive ball games	• Card games
• Sit-ups	• Floor exercises
• Yoga	

Activity, in general, should be paced and occur regularly every day.[4] Nurses should capitalise on the activities of daily living to facilitate activity at home and in the hospital setting; for example, encourage the older person to dry body parts vigorously.[6] Various exercises for bed, chair and standing are available.[5] Goals should always be realistic.[4,5] Some older people will need to have their heart rates monitored during exercise to ensure they do not overexert themselves.[4,7] Others will require an individually designed program because of chronic health problems.[4,8]

Reluctance to take part in activities

The aged fail to participate in available activities for many reasons. They include:

- their reaction to the public's perception of them as passive members of society;[4]
- their belief that the need for exercise diminishes with age;[4]
- an underestimation of their own capacity;[7]
- changes associated with normal ageing (e.g. progressively decreasing thyroid gland activity which slows metabolism);
- sensory losses;
- social isolation;
- limited financial resources;[7]
- lack of knowledge about exercise;
- negative attitudes about exercise.[10]

The elderly, in one study,[16] considered that they deserved a 'rest', because they had worked hard all their lives.

Promoting and maintaining physical integrity

Considering the barriers to activity, special efforts are needed to promote and maintain an active state in old age. Education will play an important role.[7] Healthcraft programs for those aged 50 and over are conducted in various community health centres and include such topics as 'Fitness at any Age' and 'Gentle Exercise'. Various literature is produced by the National Heart Foundation of Australia. A handbook, *Getting On*, is distributed free through community health centres and contains a major chapter on exercise. Physical activity programs will need to concentrate on marketing the health and social benefits of such programs.[16] Where the elderly are reluctant to take exercise because of various medical conditions, a separate educational program is needed. This should be conducted through an authoritative medical source (e.g. community health centre or Health Department) and advocate the use of exercise to help overcome and prevent debilitating problems.[16]

A press release by John Brown, the Minister for Sport, Recreation and Tourism, announced in 1983 that the Australian Sports Commission would investigate the sporting and recreational needs of the elderly. Among other things, they would consider the adequacy of the facilities available and the need to improve and expand those facilities. Obviously, this approach would greatly assist in improving the overall health of all Australians as well as reducing demands on the health system.[30]

Mental activity

Mental activity is as vital to the total well-being of the elderly as physical activity.[7] Stimulation and challenge help older people maintain normal mental functioning. Generally, the need for stimulation and challenge will remain consistent throughout an individual's lifetime and into old age.[7,31] Old age may also allow the individual to develop new hobbies and interests, having been freed from occupational responsibilities by retirement. Generally, the greater the level of education attained earlier in life, the more willing and likely the older person is to participate in further learning, such as adult education courses.[5,32]

It seems clear from the literature on intelligence that the elderly are capable of being mentally active even into ripe old age.[33,34] Naylor and Harwood,[35] for example, found that the involvement of aged people in the study of German led to 'extraordinary vitalising effects', including 'an increase in alertness and concentration, a broadening of horizons, a sense of group acceptance, and sheer exhilaration at the new feeling of achievement'.[36]

Older people do seem to need more time, however, to integrate new learning and to rehearse it before it is set in long-term memory. They learn more effectively when given ample time to take in and retrieve information.[37] They are also more likely to learn when the information has personal meaning for them.[33] Visual and auditory material presented at the same time will enhance learning.[33]

Developing skills

Education may assist many of the elderly to 'acquire career development and job search techniques, to acquire new and marketable skills or retool old ones, and to explore new options for earning money'.[38] New and appropriate leisure skills could be discovered by attending various craft or special interest courses (see Chapter 11). The removal of the time constraints of work can allow the older person to begin to develop unused or unknown talents and interests and thus derive great pleasure from new activities.[33,39] If older people continue to grow and develop, then they will be 'far better able to survive, to cope and to give, and will be liberated from stereotypes that limit their view of what they can accomplish'[33] (p96)

New learning may also be helpful in empowering older people to cope with mounting social and economic problems. For example, the Foster Grandparent Program in the United States enables the elderly to offer a service to children and the community and at the same time benefit emotionally from the experience.[33]

Education can help the aged to exert some degree of influence over various aspects of society which impinge on their lives.[5,33] They can become active in the political arena, for example, much like any other interest group ('Gray Panthers' in the United States and VOTE in Australia).[40]

Of the elderly that do participate in education, the primary reasons given in one study were to expand general knowledge, make good use of time, and be with others. Peterson[33] found that the aged are interested in religion, health, financial affairs, history, contemporary events, travel, arts, craft, bridge and gardening. Any activity that allows individuals to improve their skills would be useful in the satisfaction of what Crandall[5] calls transcendental needs.

Summary

Good nutrition in old age is essential for the maintenance of health, a sense of well-being and resistance to disease. This will require an adequate intake of all the essential nutrients. To achieve this, various physical, physiological and psychosocial changes associated with old age will need to be overcome by good nursing care. In some cases, an inadequate adherence to good dietary habits will need correction.

Both physical and mental activity are vital to the well-being of the elderly. Those who have been physically and mentally active all their life will have the most positive attitude towards activity in old age. Physical activity has both active and passive aspects, and should occur regularly every day. The barriers which prevent many elderly people from being active may be overcome by education, appropriate programs, and literature.

Mental stimulation and challenge will help elderly people to maintain normal mental functioning into old age. They may require more time to learn new material, but education has many advantages. It will help the elderly to continue to grow as individuals and to cope with mounting social and economic problems.

Questions

1. What is the influence of nutrition on longevity?
2. Discuss the social nature of food for the older person.
3. 'There is no evidence that requirements for nutrients decrease with age.' Discuss this statement.
4. Why is obesity such an important problem in old age?
5. Describe the social, physical and physiological factors that contribute to dietary problems in old age.
6. How may the nurse gain an accurate understanding of an older person's dietary status?
7. Why is it important that the older person's diet be individualised?

8. What practical actions can the older person take to minimise food costs and enhance dietary intake?
9. What are the benefits of physical and mental activity in old age?
10. Discuss the proposition that those who were physically and mentally active all their life tend to remain so into old age.
11. Under what circumstances will the older person qualify only for passive exercises?
12. Describe why many of the elderly do not participate in physical and mental activities.
13. How may physical and mental activity be promoted in old age?
14. What evidence is available to support the notion that the elderly are capable of learning new material?
15. How may education be helpful in old age?

Tasks

1. Ask a well older person, living in an independent situation, to keep a diary of what they eat and when they eat it, over a week. Compare the results with what you know about nutritional needs in old age.
2. Design an appropriate physical activity program for a group of
   (a) bed-bound older patients; or
   (b) well, elderly clients; or
   (c) confused elderly patients in a large hospital ward.
3. Visit an educational program for seniors, such as School for Seniors, and ascertain and evaluate the program offered.

References

1. Combs KL. Preventive care in the elderly. American Journal of Nursing August, 1978; 1333-1341.
2. Ford B. The elderly Australian. Australia: Penguin Books, 1979.
3. Ory MG. Promotion strategies for the aged. Journal of Gerontology 1985; 10(10): 31-35.
4. Ebersole P, Hess P. Toward healthy aging. St Louis: C.V. Mosby, 1985.
5. Crandall RC. Gerontology: a behavioural science approach. Reading, Massachusetts: Addison-Wesley Publishing Co. 1980.
6. Banks G. Options: a handbook for the elderly and those who care for them. Victoria, Australia: Dove Communications, 1984.
7. Eliopoulos C. Geriatric nursing. London: Harper & Row, 1980.
8. Carnevali DL, Patrick M. Nursing management for the elderly. Philadelphia: J.B. Lippincott Co. 1979.
9. Carotenuto R, Bullock J. Physical assessment of the gerontologic client. Philadelphia: F.A. Davis Co. 1981.
10. Wantz MS, Gay JE. The aging process. Cambridge, Massachusetts: Winthrop Publishers Inc. 1981.
11. Bozian MW. Nutrition for the aged or aged nutrition? Nursing Clinics of North America 1976; 11(1): 169-177.
12. Kart CS, Metress ES, Metress JF. Aging and health: biologic and social perspectives. Menlo Park, California: Addison-Wesley Publishing Co. 1978.
13. Burnside IM. Nursing and the aged. New York: McGraw-Hill Book Co. 1976.
14. Weber H. Nursing care of the elderly. Reston, Virginia: Reston Publishing Co. 1980.
15. Rowe JW, Besdine RW. Health and disease in old age. Boston: Little, Brown & Co. 1982.
16. Department of Health, NSW. Determining senior adults' needs for exercise programs: a health and leisure survey. North Ryde, NSW: Department of Health, 1984.
17. Kendig H. Housing and living arrangements of the aged. In Howe AL, ed. Towards an older Australia. Queensland, Australia: University of Queensland Press, 1981
18. Wilson HS, Kneisl CR. Psychiatric nursing. Menlo Park, California: Addison-Wesley Publishing Co. 1985.
19. Howe AL, ed. Towards an older Australia. Queensland, Australia: University of Queensland Press, 1981.
20. Russell C. The aging experience. London: George Allen & Unwin, 1981.
21. Prinsley D. Research perspectives. In Howe AL, ed. Towards an older Australia. Queensland, Australia: University of Queensland Press, 1981.
22. NSW Council on the Ageing Migrant Advisory Committee. Where to next? Sydney, Australia: The NSW Council on the Ageing Ltd, 1983.
23. Johnson-Pawlson J, Koshes R. Exercise is for everyone. Gerontological Nursing 1985; 6(6): 322-325.
24. Parent CJ, Whall AJ. Are physical activity, self-esteem, and depression related? Journal of Gerontological Nursing 1984; 10(9): 8-11.
25. Bassett C, McClamrock E, Schmelzer M. A ten-week exercise program for senior citizens. Geriatric Nursing March/April 1982; 103-105.
26. Clark BA, Wade MG, Massey BH, Van Dyke R. Response of institutionalised geriatric mental patients to a twelve-week programme of regular physical activity. Journal of Gerontology 1975; 30(5): 565-573.

27. de Vries HA. Physiology of exercise and aging. In Woodruff DS, Birren JE, eds. Aging: scientific perspectives and social issues. New York: Van Nostrand Reinhold Co. 1975.
28. Goldberg WG, Fitzpatrick JL. Movement therapy with the aged. Nursing Research 1980; 29: 339.
29. Comfort A. A good age. North Sydney: Macmillan, 1977.
30. Press release, John Brown, Federal Minister for Sport, Recreation and Tourism (Australia), 22 September, 1983.
31. Murray R, Huelskoetter MM, O'Driscoll D. The nursing process in later maturity. Englewood Cliffs, New Jersey: Prentice-Hall Inc. 1980.
32. Botwinick J. Aging and behaviour. New York: Springer, 1978.
33. Peterson DA. Facilitating education for older learners. San Francisco: Jossey-Bass, 1983.
34. Knox AB. New direction for continuing education. Assessing the impact of continuing education. No. 3. San Francisco: Jossey-Bass, 1979.
35. Naylor G, Harwood E. Old dogs, new tricks: age and ability. Psychology Today 1975; 1(1): 16, 29-33.
36. Harwood E. The learning capacities of the aging. Social Sciences 1971; 22(5): 1,2-5.
37. Bolton EB. Cognitive and non-cognitive factors that affect learning in older adults and their implications for instruction. Educational Gerontology 1978; 3: 331-334.
38. Lowry L. Continuing education in the later years: learning in the third age. Gerontology and Geriatrics Education 1983; 4(2): 95.
39. Kerschner L, Kerschner P. A difference of opinion on higher education and the elderly. Gerontology and Geriatrics Education 1982; 3(2): 121-128.
40. Harris L and Associates. The myth and reality of aging in America. Washington, DC: National Council of the Aging, 1975.

Chapter 4

Communicating with the Older Person

Objectives

To enable the reader to:

1. define the term communication;
2. identify the elements in the communication process;
3. list and briefly describe the different types of communication;
4. identify physical and psychosocial barriers to communication;
5. discuss how communication with older patients and clients may be made more effective;
6. describe the usefulness of touch in older patient and client care;
7. appreciate the need to provide time for solitude for older patients.

Before the introduction of the Nursing Process, patients' needs were assessed in terms of the 'medical model' and not necessarily by nurses caring for the patient. Procedures were by-and-large standardised for all patients.[1] Thus, all patients had temperature, pulse, respiration and blood pressure charted regularly, but only some had other procedures carried out on them. Such standardisation had its uses but some patients received unwelcome attentions which were perhaps unnecessary. Nursing was also characterised by task allocation rather than patient allocation; this often led to depersonalised care because task allocation emphasised physical care to meet physical needs.

The introduction of the Nursing Process, which made assessment of the patient's or client's needs a nursing responsibility, moved nursing away from the medical model to more personalised, problem-based care.[2] It is not difficult to see that the new approach requires something totally different from the nurse in terms of attitudes towards patient care.

The most basic skill involved will be that of communication.[3] The ability to communicate is vital if the nurse is to make a proper assessment of older patients' needs. Evaluating their needs should be made on the basis of a nursing history. For this, the nurse must not only be able to communicate well but must also be skilled in interviewing techniques (see Chapter 6). In addition, nursing assessment will include an assessment of sight and sound acuity, voice quality, and the functioning of the tongue, teeth, pharynx and larynx. The level of the patient's ability to read, write and understand the spoken language should also be ascertained.[4]

In this chapter, communication is examined in relation to the nursing process.

Communication

Schramm[5] has pointed out that the word 'communication' comes from the Latin *communis*, meaning 'common'. When we communicate, therefore, we are trying to establish a 'commonness' with someone else, that is, we are trying to share information, or an idea, or perhaps an attitude (see also Cohen, in Sundeen *et al*, 1976). It is not a one-way ('linear') activity but an interactional or two-way process.[6] In any communication transaction, both participants are communicators.

According to Yearwood-Grazette,[7] there are five elements in the process or act of communication:

1. a communicator
2. a message
3. a code
4. a channel
5. a receiver

I feel this list is incomplete and would prefer to add three more elements so that the process looks like this:

1. a communicator
2. the encoding process
3. a message
4. a code
5. a channel

6. a receiver
7. the decoding process
8. feedback or checking out

A communicator (1) is an individual or group who transmits a message (3). The message refers to the meaning to be communicated. The communicator has a mental perception of what he/she wishes to send. This idea is translated (2) into a code that will enable it to be transmitted to someone else. The code (4) may be verbal, non-verbal or written. The code is the particular way in which the message is to be delivered which is understandable to both the sender and receiver of the message. English is an appropriate code for many Australians although this situation is changing rapidly. The channel (5) I have been using in this chapter is that of writing, but others, such as drawing, are also available.

The use of the term 'receiver' (6) is somewhat misleading as it seems to imply a passive role in terms of action or response. But the receiver must be able to receive and decode the message (7) being transmitted, to give it meaning. It may be difficult for a deaf person, or someone suffering from the later stages of Alzheimer's disease, to receive and decode a message transmitted verbally. Similarly, older people who are blind will not be able to 'pick up' non-verbal cues, such as facial expression.

Interpretation and understanding of the message (7) will depend on a number of variables, including the congruence of verbal and non-verbal communication (whether what is actually being said is reinforced or contradicted by body language or other non-verbal cues). If the communication has been effective, an alteration in behaviour should follow. This does not necessarily mean, however, that the receiver will choose to behave in the manner predicted by the sender of the message. Feedback (8) from the receiver will indicate the degree of understanding achieved and complete the communication cycle.

Types of communication

These include:

- written
- verbal
- non-verbal
- meta-communication

Verbal communication represents 'an amazing conceptualisation of symbols which put together form language'.[8] It requires the use of spoken words and a knowledge of the language.[2] Numerous non-verbal behaviour channels exist. They include tone of voice, posture, gesture, body movements, body contact, facial expression and movements (including gaze and eye contact), touch, the use of space, the use of time, and appearance and clothes.[3,8,9] Many researchers agree that these channels carry more social meaning then verbal ones.[6] Non-verbal messages, then, are often a more reliable indicator of real meaning in communication than what is said, because they are not under such conscious control.[10] Information about emotions or feelings is usually transmitted more accurately in non-verbal fashion.

Meta-communication occurs at both the verbal and non-verbal levels. It is basically communication about communication.[9] It has been defined by Satir[11] as a 'comment on the literal content as well as on the nature of the relationship between the persons involved'. It conveys, therefore, the sender's attitude towards himself, the message and the listener. Meta-communication can be seen where the nurse conveys by various means (e.g. overly 'fussing around' the patient, over-concern or excessive attention) the fact that something is seriously amiss. This is perceived by the patient as: 'Something is wrong, but they're keeping me in the dark.'

Communicating with the elderly

For the elderly in particular, we must provide opportunities for continual interpersonal relationships even though at times these may be difficult to maintain because of disease and we may feel inept in the situation. One of the most important goals of the nurse-older person relationship is the establishment of therapeutic interpersonal relationships.[4] The role of the nurse as communicator will involve listening, initiating, developing and maintaining relationships with the older person so as to help them to maintain maximum contact with others in their environment.

The art of communicating with the elderly person may at times require short, simple messages. Sometimes the initial interaction will begin with questions about their present problems; this may lead on to discussion about their past life and accomplishments and current problems generally. The nurse can build on these initial interactions to begin to form a relationship with the older person in which deeper issues can be discussed.

A thorough assessment of the older person's communication capabilities may help to identify potentially treatable conditions. Assessment will include the older person's perceptual status, the anatomical apparatus associated with speech production, and an appraisal of the ability to read, write and understand spoken language.[4]

Barriers to communication in old age

These have been divided into physical and psychosocial barriers. Physical barriers include:

- physical disability (e.g. deafness and blindness);

- physical discomfort (e.g. temperature, ventilation, pain, urge to micturate);
- illness (e.g. organic brain syndrome, cerebrovascular accident);
- time of day;
- noise and interruptions (e.g. phone, other people);
- being too busy to spend time with the older person.

Deafness may exist in varying degrees in old age, from a slight hearing difficulty to total deafness. The aged may not always realise that their hearing is defective,[12] so this may be a serious problem with elderly people. Hearing defects may be caused by cerumen, otosclerosis and presbycussis.[13] Hearing difficulties in older people are highly significant and may lead the older adult to become isolated, bad-tempered, aggressive, angry, depressed, confused or even paranoid. Problems of deafness may be handled in several ways. These include:

- raising the voice moderately, and enunciating clearly and slowly while facing the older person;
- using written forms of communication;
- finding other words to say the same thing;
- using non-verbal communication to enhance verbal messages;
- encouraging the hearing-impaired older person to remain socially active;
- reducing the competition from extraneous sounds when talking with the hearing-impaired person;
- encouraging the older person to use a hearing aid.

Difficulty in speaking varies from a slight slowing down of speech to aphasia.[13] Generally, the voice loses strength and volume and becomes slower with age.[13] Pathological changes may occur, including abnormality in the neuromuscular function of the lips, tongue, palate, vocal cords, or the muscles of respiration.[14] Depression may also develop. Ill-fitting dentures or poor oral hygiene which is sufficient to interfere with tongue movements may also be implicated.[15]

It becomes crucial in aged care that full use of alternatives to speech is achieved and maintained, especially for those older people with long-term speech difficulties. Carnevali and Patrick[16] have identified a number of these alternatives:

- pointing, gestures and pantomime;
- cards with common requests or words;
- encouraging non-verbal activities with others so that they can feel self-worth and companionship.

Difficulty in understanding. The older person may be less alert and forget more easily, especially recent events. They may be slow to understand the meaning of words. These problems are sometimes covered up by the older people themselves or by their relatives. Difficulties in understanding may be related to the presence of organic brain syndrome, confusion, depression, cerebrovascular disease[17] and many other problems. Other causes include cultural and language differences.

Visual defects block communication at any age, but in the elderly the problem becomes more severe because of other losses that are occurring at the same time. An initial eye examination and then annual examinations are extremely important. Visual deficits may result from cataracts, glaucoma, senile macular degeneration or cerebrovascular disease.[13]

Psychosocial barriers to communication with the older person are many and varied and it is important that they are recognised. They include:

- the effects of ascribed and assumed roles (e.g. the nurse may be seen as an authority figure by the older person, and the nurse accepts this role and acts accordingly towards the older person);
- the influence of unconscious and partly conscious mechanisms (including all the methods the mind employs to select and distort the material received so that it fits the self-concept of the receiver);[9]
- lack of motivation on the part of the nurse or older person;
- the older person's emotional state (they may be anxious, depressed, scared);[4]
- educational differences between the older person and the nurse, including different learning styles;
- prejudices held by the nurse towards older people;
- the presence of frank psychiatric illness (e.g. dementia, paranoid illness, manic-depressive psychosis).

Cultural barriers to effective communication include language differences and the beliefs and values of the older person and the nurse. Barriers to communication may also be related to the socioeconomic status and intelligence levels of the nurse and the older patient.[10]

Communication with older people may not always be reciprocal, that is, you may sometimes have to continue without very much response. In such situations it is easy to become discouraged but such feelings should be controlled. If the nurse makes them apparent, these feelings may reinforce the older person's existing anxieties and cause them to feel more insecure and anxious, thus interfering further with the communication process. Talking to other colleagues about this situation may help you with your own feelings and enable you to respond more positively to the older person's needs.[18]

The nurse may contribute to problems in the communication process by not organising her thoughts before communicating; including too many ideas at once; not giving the older person her full attention when communicating; thinking about her own replies rather than what the older person is saying; and listening for details rather than the essential message. To this list Murray, Huelskoetter and O'Driscoll[18] have added other problems arising from the nurse-older person relationship. These include:

- feeling that you are the only nurse who can help the older person;
- becoming involved with the older person as a friend and so losing objectivity;
- using intimidation to control the older person;
- probing and challenging the older person;
- interrupting, speaking too loudly;
- using patronising behaviour, including verbal communication.

Evaluating nurse-older person communication

It should be obvious by now that many things can go wrong in the communication process involving the older person and the nurse. Cohen[9] has provided a structure against which communication may be evaluated. The elements involved include the effectiveness, appropriateness, adequacy, efficiency and flexibility of the communication (see also Wilson and Kneisl, 1985).[6]

Effectiveness determines how successful the communication is in meeting the goals of the interaction. A common problem in evaluating effectiveness, however, is subjectivity. To obviate this it is necessary to have preplanned behavioural goals against which to measure the behavioural outcomes of the interaction.

Appropriateness refers to the relevancy of the communication in meeting the desired outcomes. It takes into account the uniqueness of the participation and the context or time of the interaction.

Adequacy refers to the amount of communication used to reach the desired goal. Is there sufficient communication to accomplish the purpose? Has sufficient feedback been received, acknowledged and accurately interpreted?

Efficient communication uses direct and simple language and instructions are clear and agreed upon.

The last criterion for successful communication is flexibility. Rigid approaches in which the nurse attempts to control the interaction are not helpful. They prevent the nurse from knowing the older person as a unique individual because the patient is relegated to the status of an object. Permissiveness will help the older person to maintain independent decision making.

Effective communication

The nurse as communicator 'listens, and initiates, develops, and maintains relationships that can effectively aid in the maintenance of the health of the individual, family and community'.[4] Of all the subjects in nursing syllabi, communication and communication skills are perhaps the most difficult areas to teach and develop.[19]

Various forms of behaviour have been found to be effective in promoting effective communication in the nurse-older person relationship.[4,8,10,20] These techniques include:

- facing the older person squarely when communicating;
- adopting an open posture;
- leaning towards the older person if seated;
- keeping good eye contact;
- maintaining the same eye level as the older person;
- concentrating on the older person and what they say;
- being relaxed;
- using touch therapeutically;
- using open-ended questions to encourage the older person to 'open up';
- trying to listen with understanding; that is, trying to see the expressed idea/s and attitude/s from the older person's point of view.

Responding to the older person with respect, genuineness and warmth are also desirable behaviours.[6] Kron[10] has provided a useful set of 'keys' to effective communication. Obviously, these must be used continually if we are to understand others and be understood by them. The keys are:

- Understand your own ideas before you try to pass them on;
- Use the right word in the right place to the right person at the right time in the right manner;
- Don't forget to look for and evaluate feedback;
- Allow other people to express their ideas;
- Observe! Observe! Observe!;
- Seek not only to be understood but to understand.

Promises to older people should not be broken and relevant information should be provided when asked for. They should not be told 'what to do'.[8] The older person's feelings should be readily acknowledged[21] and should not be reacted to with clichés and glib remarks.[22]

Empathy, congruence and positive regard are thus integral aspects of therapeutic communication. Carkhuff[23] developed scales to measure the dimensions of these concepts in interpersonal situations other than counselling. These, in turn, were adapted by Aspy[24] to examine the nurse educator-student nurse relationship. The purpose was to identify nurse educator behaviours which the nursing students perceived as empathic, congruent and having positive regard. I have adapted these findings here because these behaviours are also effective if adopted by the nurse in the nurse-older person relationship (see Table 4.1).

Table 4.1 Effective Nurse Behaviours in Older Person Relationships

Empathy	**Congruence**	**Positive regard**
• shows understanding	• shares self	• gives positive feedback
• sees older person as an individual	• will admit mistakes	• trusts older person
• has realistic expectations of the older person	• is willing to evaluate self	• respects older person
• cares about the older person	• is human	• is receptive to older person
• knows the older person	• acknowledges the older person	• willing to listen to the older person
• is supportive	• can accept criticism	• promotes interaction and older person involvement in the care program
• is sensitive to the older person	• can achieve and maintain a personalised relationship	
• is willing to help	• is honest	• treats older person as an intelligent individual
• remembers that she will also be old one day and will experience illness and hospitalisation		

Touch

Whenever we become aware of others, our world expands beyond ourselves to include relationships with others. This is the beginning of the process of communication. One of the first and most fundamental means of communicating with others is through some form of touch.[25] Touch conveys meaning and the particular meaning conveyed is often culture-bound.[8] In all human cultures physical contact plays an important role in interpersonal relations.

The familiar sense of touch is not a single sense but includes pressure, pain, warmth and cold, all felt through distinct kinds of sensitive spots on the skin surfaces. The normal adult skin has millions of these receptors.[10] All other sensations are variations of the four senses identified.

Neurologically, touch is conducted by the central nervous system fibres that are myelinated earliest in the foetus.[26] The earliest and most fundamental medium of human communication, then, is touch.[25,27-29] The foetus experiences:

- warm contact in the womb;
- rhythmic impact of the maternal heartbeats;
- contractions of the uterus during birth;
- contact with the vaginal canal during birth;
- the obstetrician's or midwife's hands.

Much of the infant's early communication is also by touch. The infant, for example, is:

- patted and cuddled;
- breast-fed;
- handled often, fed, bathed and changed.

Through these experiences the child begins to establish and maintain intercourse with the world around it. Denial or deprivation of these early tactile experiences may seriously impair the child's future ability to learn,[23] to establish loving relationships, to communicate with others generally[28] and to maintain internal homeostasis.[29]

Research studies

Not until the 1950s did studies begin to appear reporting systematic attempts to transcribe gestures and other non-verbal behaviours.[25] Since the 1950s there have been an increasing number of studies which have focused on touch as a non-verbal means of communication.

There have been some studies of the effective use of touch with patients. Being touched frequently was found by de Augustus *et al*[30] to decrease the anxiety of patients. Earlier, Charlton[31] concluded from her studies that when the nurse interprets the symbolic verbal and non-verbal behaviour of the patient as a request for physical contact, the patient 'moves' towards the nurse. Burnside,[32] working with six regressed aged persons, discovered that a warm, simple, human gesture, like a hand on the shoulder, helped to make them respond more than many sophisticated techniques. To investigate the effects of touch on non-verbal communication, on seriously ill patients, McCorkle[27] demonstrated that the nurse can establish a rapport with a seriously ill patient within a short time. Adult critically ill patients, with stable but not necessarily normal vital signs, were studied by Knable[33] for the effects of hand-holding by nurses on their psychophysiological responses. Findings supported the use of hand-holding as a therapeutic nursing intervention. Langland and Panicucci[34] found that touch increased responses in the elderly confused.

The use of touch in nursing

When admitted to hospital, older people often become dependent on those who care for them. Also, hospitalisation often involves a reduction in contact with the outside world.[27,28] This may also be the case even when the older person is living at home and being visited by the community nurse. In these situations, patients may resort to earlier modes of interaction to handle situations which arise. These may not always be successful or appropriate, and touch may help to re-establish normal relationships with others.

Touch is perhaps one of the more important expressions of communication in the nurse-older person relationship. One cannot imagine nursing being performed without touch,[26] for nurses are designated 'touchers' by virtue of their profession.[28] Although we learn to socialise our need for touch, under certain conditions such as illness or stress we may temporarily return to the basic needs of our earlier days. Older people are more prone to illness and multiple stresses, suggesting an increased need for caring physical contact from those responsible for caring for them.[29] They may also have a greater need for touch because of decreased perceptual capacities, such as vision and hearing. Loss of friends and loved ones makes touch more significant with increasing age.

The technique of touch consists of the simple placing of the hands for 10 to 15 minutes on or close to the body of the older patient by the person who intends to help or heal them.[26] This physical contact may take many forms. These include shaking hands, a hand on the shoulder, dancing, patting hands, joining hands, hugging, general massage, holding hands firmly, stroking the arm or forehead.[26,29,32] It is important to be willing to allow the older person to touch you too.

The therapeutic effects of touch

Hardy[35] believes that touch can relieve the special anxieties and concerns of the older person. It provides opportunities for a mutual exchange of trust and sharing in situations of intense personal stress, such as hospitalisation. No other way of communicating can compare 'in immediacy to the comforting and quieting effects of touch'.[27] Moreover, touch:

- demonstrates concern and caring;[32,35,36]
- reassures older people who have had major surgery, which has led to some degree of disfigurement, that they are still lovable;[26]
- calms and soothes;[32]
- conveys to the older person that he is not alone;[37]
- reduces and relieves physical and psychological pain;[25,28]
- conveys a sense of general acceptance;[29]
- provides comfort in dying.[27]

Touch can be very therapeutic but should not be used where it causes the nurse herself discomfort. Conversely, the nurse should be alert to any discomfort caused to the older person by the nurse's use of touch. Apart from these caveats, touch when used with care and sensitivity can be especially therapeutic for the aged person.

Providing time for solitude

Although the nurse aims at all times to keep communication open between the older person and herself and others, there is also a need to provide time for solitude for the older person so that decision making, reflecting, reminiscing and thinking will not be continually interrupted by others. Perhaps designated areas should be provided for such purposes, especially in hospitals and nursing homes. Nurses must be sensitive to this need, but must also carefully assess the degree of solitude and social interaction and help to maintain a balance of both.[38]

Summary

The introduction of the Nursing Process requires that the nurse be able to communicate effectively. When we communicate we try to establish a 'commonness' with the other person. Communication may be verbal or non-verbal. Barriers to communication exist, both physical and psychosocial, but therapeutic nursing interventions can reduce these problems. The use of touch is often helpful in caring for the older person, and the provision of time for solitude is necessary.

Questions

1. What is communication?
2. List and describe briefly the eight elements involved in the process of communication.
3. What is non-verbal communication?
4. Why is touch a helpful form of communication in geriatric nursing?
5. Explain how the nurse's emotional state can act as a barrier to effective communication.

6. What is the relationship between 'keeping promises' and effective communication?
7. How may the geriatric nurse communicate more effectively?
8. Describe positive nurse behaviours in therapeutic communication, using the following headings:
   (a) empathy
   (b) congruence
   (c) positive regard.

Discussion task

Describe and analyse any two effective and any two ineffective communication processes which you have been involved in or observed, in a ward or community nursing situation.

Case study

A 65-year-old woman, Mrs Collins, with right-sided hemiplegia, lives in her own home and receives visits every two days from the community nurse. Her family is fairly supportive and her daughter in particular visits or phones every day. Her life has been a hard one and her marriage of 25 years was not very happy. She has been a widow for five years. She does not respond very often when addressed by the community nurse.

Mrs Collins has had hemiplegia for two years, and for six months of that time she was in a rehabilitation unit. There she learned to dress (if someone helped with buttons and zippers) and feed herself and transfer from her wheelchair to commode and bed.

Recently, she was admitted by her family doctor to a nursing home. In the nursing home she is not:

- receiving adequate nursing care;
- receiving adequate physical therapy;
- communicating with staff or family members when they come to visit.

For discussion

(a) What factors might have contributed to Mrs Collins' present non-communicative state?

(b) How would you as a nurse, working in the nursing home, establish and maintain communication?

References

1. Faulkner A. Aye, there's the rub. Nursing Times Feb. 1981; 19: 332-336.
2. Bridge W. and Clark J. Communication in nursing. Nursing Times 1 Jan. 1981; 1063-1064.
3. Burlew C. Communication and nursing. The Australian Nurses Journal 1981; 11(2): 41-42.
4. Ebersole P, Hess P. Toward healthy aging. St Louis: C.V. Mosby, 1981.
5. Schramm W, Roberts DF, eds. The process and effects of mass communication. Urbane: University of Illinois Press, 1974.
6. Wilson HS, Kneisl CR. Psychiatric nursing. 2nd ed. California, Menlo Park: Addison-Wesley, 1983.
7. Yearwood-Grazette HS. An anatomy of communication. Nursing Times 12 Oct. 1978; 1672-1678.
8. Porritt L. Communication for nurses. Melbourne: Churchill Livingstone, 1984.
9. Cohen SP. Communication. In Sundeen SJ et al, eds. Nurse-client interaction. Implementing the nursing process. St Louis: C.V. Mosby, 1976.
10. Kron T. Communication in nursing. Philadelphia: W.B. Saunders Co. 1972.
11. Satir V. Conjoint family therapy. Rev. Ed. Palo Alto, California: Science & Behaviour Books, 1967.
12. Stevens MK. Geriatric nursing for practical nurses. Philadelphia: W.B. Saunders, 1975.
13. Libow LS, Sherman FT. The core of geriatric medicine. St Louis: C.V. Mosby, 1981.
14. Weber HI, Nursing care of the elderly. Reston, Virginia: Prentice-Hall Co. 1980.
15. Ham R, Holtzman JM, Marcy ML, Smith MR. Primary care geriatrics. Boston: John Wright, 1983.
16. Carnevali NL, Patrick M. Nursing management for the elderly. Philadelphia: J.B. Lippincott Co. 1979.
17. Loader A. A good gossip goes a long way. Nursing Mirror 8 Jan. 1981; 34-35.
18. Murray R, Huelskoetter MM, O'Driscoll D. The nursing process in later maturity. Englewood Cliffs, New Jersey: Prentice-Hall Inc. 1980.

19. Lawson K. Listening to patients. Nursing Times 9 Oct. 1980; 1784-1788.
20. Sundeen SJ et al. Nurse-client interaction. St Louis: C.V. Mosby, 1976.
21. Ashton K. Scenes from nursing life. 2. Price and prejudice. Nursing Times 27 Jan. 1982; 161-162.
22. Iveson-Iveson J. The art of communication. Nursing Mirror Feb. 1983; 47-48.
23. Carkhuff RR. Helping and human relations. New York: Holt, Rinehart and Winston, 1969.
24. Aspy D. Toward a technology for humanising education. In Karns PJ, Schwab TA. Therapeutic communication and clinical instruction. Nursing Outlook Jan. 1982; 39-43.
25. Barnett K. A theoretical construct of the concepts of touch as they relate to nursing. Nursing Research 1972; 21(2): 102-110.
26. Krieger D. Therapeutic touch: the imprimateur of nursing. American Journal of Nursing May 1975; 785-787.
27. McCorkle R. Effects of touch on seriously ill patients. Nursing Research 1974; 23(2): 125-132.
28. Mason A, Pratt J. Touch. Nursing Times 5 June 1980: 999-1001.
29. Seaman L. Affective nursing touch. Geriatric Nursing May/June 1982; 162-164.
30. de Augustus et al. In Barnett K. A theoretical construct of the concepts of touch as they relate to nursing. Nursing Research 1972; 21(2): 102-110.
31. Charlton A. In Barnett K. A theoretical construct of the concepts of touch as they relate to nursing. Nursing Research 1972; 21(2): 102-110.
32. Burnside IM. Touch is talking. American Journal of Nursing Dec. 1983; 2060-2063.
33. Knable J. Handholding: one means of transcending barriers of communication. Heart & Lung 1981; 10(6): 1106-1110.
34. Langland RM, Panicucci CL. Effects of touch on communication with elderly confused clients. Journal of Gerontological Nursing 1982; 8(3): 152-155.
35. Hardy J. The importance of touch for patient and nurse. The Journal of Practical Nursing June 1975; 26-27.
36. Amacher NJ. Touch is a way of caring. American Journal of Nursing May 1983; 852-854.
37. de Thomaso MT. 'Touch power' and the screen of loneliness. The Lamp Feb. 1982; 14-17.
38. Eliopoulos C. Geriatric nursing. London: Harper & Row, 1980.

Chapter 5

The Aged of non-English-speaking Background in Australia

Objectives

To enable the reader to:

1. appreciate that the ethnic aged are not a homogeneous group with common needs;
2. describe specific problems experienced by ageing migrants of non-English-speaking background;
3. discuss the role of the nurse in relation to the ethnic aged;
4. identify the need for more research.

Since World War II, Australia's population has grown from about 7 million to 16 million in the late 1980s. A great proportion of this population increase is due to Australia's major migration program, directed at encouraging settlers, initially from European, later from Middle Eastern, Asian and South American countries.

Throughout the 1950-1960 period it was assumed that immigrants would and should adapt to the established social norms and values (Assimilationist Policy). Accordingly, government policy in service delivery continued on the model of 'assimilative and universal service delivery'. It assumed a shared value system and made no particular attempt to identify and respond to the cultural experience (and linguistic barriers) of immigrants, to enable them to gain access to these mainstream services.[1]

Analysis of service usage pattern, however, showed that people of non-English-speaking origin were proportionately under-represented among service users and, if they did gain access to services, it was usually in crisis situations only.

In response to an increasingly pluralist society, Australia in the 1970s adopted the philosophical position of 'multiculturalism'. Multiculturalism accepts cultural and linguistic differences and has three aims: social cohesion; cultural identity; and equality of opportunity and access.[2]

Various legislation has been introduced, both at Commonwealth and State government levels, to overcome obstacles to equal access and equity (e.g. the Racial Discrimination Act; Equal Employment Opportunity legislation; the NSW Anti-Discrimination Act). In the 1980s the New South Wales Government introduced the policy of 'mainstreaming' services; that is, mainstream services would be diversified to meet more effectively the variety of needs in a pluralist society:

> Mainstreaming has developed out of a perceived shift of responsibility in the delivery of services, away from the client and to the service provider. This can be seen as the public policy implication of the historical shift from the policies of assimilation to the principles of multiculturalism. Peter Sheldrake, the director of the Australian Institute of Multicultural Affairs, in a presentation on mainstreaming coined it thus: 'Under an assimilationist policy it is the migrants who are mainstreamed; multiculturalism mainstreams the services.'[3]

The policy to mainstream services followed a review by the Ethnic Affairs Commission of New South Wales of the State Government's ethnic affairs policy and implementation achievements over recent years. It found that, while many specialist ethnic affairs units within public administrations provided valuable services, these were often marginalised and not seen as part of the mainstream functions.

Thus in 1984 state departments and authorities were required to develop 'Ethnic Affairs Policy Statements' (EAPS) based on the following principles:

- the right of equality of access to services regardless of cultural origin or linguistic skills;
- the responsibility of service providers to respond appropriately to their target population, which included people of non-English-speaking background.

Similarly, the Commonwealth Government has developed draft guidelines on 'Access and Equity' to encourage Commonwealth and Local Government services to respond more effectively to the needs of ethnic communities in Australia.[4]

In practical terms, Liffman[1] describes this kind of service model as 'assimilative and ethnic targeted'. It assumes common needs but provides some facilitating services such as interpreters, bilingual staff and multilingual information provision to improve access to mainstream services. While this can be regarded as a first step, ethnic community organisations argue that more emphasis should be placed on evaluating service outcome; that is, their concern is that many of the available mainstream services do not meet the specific needs of immigrants in different stages in the life cycle. Indeed, former Minister of Community Services, the Hon. Don Grimes, in an address concerning mainstreaming, commented:

> Issues which ultimately have to be resolved include:
> - the most effective means of dealing with language barriers;
> - how best to address cultural, religious and dietary preferences;
> - a possible shortage of appropriately trained ethnic staff (such as nurses) to run suitable programs;
> - alternative means of providing services, such as developing a network of volunteer and/or other workers;
> - means of meeting the needs of fragmented, geographically dispersed and smaller ethnic groups.[3]

Research into the needs of older people of non-English-speaking background

Until recently little research had been conducted into the needs of older members of minority groups in predominantly industrialised, English-speaking countries. According to Crandall,[5] early gerontologists generally represented older people of other non-English-speaking cultures as a homogeneous group with common needs. Studies did not distinguish their participants by race or ethnic origin. During the 1950s (in the United States), and even later in other countries, the concept of homogeneity of the aged population began to change, and many of the factors that make the older population a heterogeneous group began to be recognised. However, even with this recognition, little research appeared until recently. Gerontologists seem to have been more interested in other areas of gerontology. Older people of non-English-speaking background may have been perceived as suspicious of research, and language may also have been a problem.

Bengtson[6] argues that one of the reasons for the scant attention social scientists have paid to the pluralist nature of the older population is that few studies into minority groups have been placed into theoretical constructs on ageing, which would allow for policy development to meet the variety of physical, social and emotional needs of a pluralist population. For example, while the physical process of ageing is likely to affect people similarly, irrespective of where they were born, their coping strategies to deal with the consequences of growing older will differ between groups. Thus, research into ethnic group differences should concentrate on issues relating to:

- the social stratification of a pluralist society;
- the size and social resources of specific ethnic groups;
- the perceived accessibility of relevant services;
- the cultural values and personal resources of the elderly to deal with everyday life.

Bengtson[6] cites several examples of recent research which explore the question of whether ethnicity *per se* makes a difference to the pattern of growing old within a pluralist society. In one study,[6] two theoretical propositions were explored. One perspective suggested that the aged in minority groups suffer from a situation of 'double jeopardy' or 'multiple hazards'. These descriptions refer to the additive negative effects of being old *and* a member of a racial or ethnic minority. The second perspective viewed advancing years as 'a leveller' of the ethnic inequalities that existed during the working life of individuals (e.g. the loss of work status upon retirement would affect people similarly in different groups, or health status may decline irrespective of country of origin).

Accordingly, variables such as income, health, life satisfaction and social interactions between different age groups of Anglo-Americans and minority groups were measured. Results showed that, in terms of relative income and health, minority elderly may indeed be characterised as experiencing 'double jeopardy'. While income declined in all respondents by age stratum, not only was the mean income lower among minority groups, it also declined more rapidly with advancing years. Similarly, ethnic minority members were significantly more likely to report poorer health than respondents of the dominant group. (The study controlled for socio-economic background within groups.)

The analysis of variables measuring life satisfaction, however, was more complex and did not clearly support either the 'double jeopardy' or the 'advancing age as leveller' hypothesis. Indicators of social interactions showed clear group differences in social network patterns. While ethnic aged had more frequent contact with their children and grandchildren than Anglo-Americans, the latter group had considerably more contact with friends, neighbours and acquaintances. These results do not support the 'double jeopardy' perspective, but they demonstrate the greater dependence among ethnic aged on their immediate family (if available).

These issues will be further discussed in the Australian context. The point Bengtson makes is that we cannot presume that ethnic differences alone are sufficient to explain the personal and social situation of the aged. To view ethnicity in isolation would ignore tremendous variation, both across ethnic boundaries and within ethnic groups. Furthermore, results depend on the kinds of aspects of the older person's life that are under study. Thus Bengtson argues that the existence of 'double jeopardy' or 'age as a leveller of inequalities' is an empirical, not a logical, question. If researched properly, however, it may give us the basis for social policy development to bring about resource allocation to meet the needs of a pluralist society. In Australia, for example, a major research study was conducted by Kendig, Gibson, Rowland and Hemer,[7] of the Ageing and the Family Project, Australian National University, to establish the factors contributing to aged people being in need of institutional care. Not surprisingly, it identified those most likely to be 'at risk' of institutionalisation as those with no spouse and/or no family members, those with low income (full age pension) and those with some disability (reduced mobility, difficulty in personal care, etc.). The study estimates that 7 per cent of all elderly people, sixty years and older, living in the community, are in 'triple jeopardy' by virtue of having all three of these substantial limitations.

More recently, the Australian Institute of Multicultural Affairs[8] has conducted major research into ethnic groups with an increasing proportion of older people. This survey shared a number of questions with the earlier study conducted by the Australian National University, which comprised mainly Anglo-Australian respondents, thus allowing for comparison between groups. Extracts follow of some of the Institute's findings on 'Community and Institutional Care for Aged Migrants in Australia'.[9]

Initially, the Institute provided these definitions and explanations. The word 'ethnic' is generally used to describe those who were born in countries where the first language spoken is not English, and who now live in Australia. The word is commonly used in this way in Australia. However, its usage in no way implies a definition of ethnic identity. It was not until the 1986 census[10] that more detailed information on ethnicity and ethnic identity was collected, and the results still await analysis. The word 'aged' refers to those who are 60 years and older. It is recognised that many people are able to lead an active life into very old age, but 60 years or more was selected mainly for practical purposes.

The ageing of ethnic communities in Australia

The proportion of people of non-English-speaking background, 60 years and older, in Australia is expected to grow from 11 per cent in 1981[11] to 22 per cent of the total aged population in 2001. The relative rapid ageing among specific ethnic groups can be explained by past migration patterns to Australia. Today's disparate demographic distribution among immigrant communities reflects the peak settlement period as well as subsequent migration patterns of particular groups. After World War II, for instance, only very limited emigration was possible from Eastern European countries, and emigration from Northern and Southern Europe peaked only in the late 1960-1970 period. Substantial intake of refugees and immigrants from Middle Eastern, Asian and South American countries did not begin until the early 1970s.

Thus an essential point to be made is that the ethnic population is not only growing, it is also changing. Some groups are clustered in very narrow age ranges and have very specific needs, as a consequence of the circumstances surrounding their original migration and settlement.

While at present the Eastern European groups have the greatest number and proportion of elderly members, the most rapid increases in the 75-plus age group in the next two decades are expected to be among those born in the Netherlands, Poland, Yugoslavia, Greece and Germany.[12]

Geographical distribution

Geographically, the ethnic aged are more concentrated in capital cities than are the Australian-born aged. Nevertheless, contrary to popular belief, individual ethnic groups are not usually concentrated in any one local area – they are dispersed throughout metropolitan regions and industrial centres in the country areas (e.g. Wollongong, Newcastle and Geelong). There may be a considerable number of elderly in the largest groups (Italian, Greek, Yugoslavs) in any given local government area, but smaller communities are also equally scattered with fewer numbers in any one area.[10]

Geographical dispersement inhibits contact between elderly of the same background, and the location of appropriate ethnic community facilities may be far removed. A report from the Polish Welfare and Information Bureau states:

> Establishing volunteer programs is very difficult where volunteers themselves are pensioners and suffer both economic limitations and restrictions to their mobility. These factors all contribute to the lack of services and complete isolation of many of the Polish aged.[13]

Geographical dispersement also affects health and welfare service provision and needs to be taken into account when planning community care as well as residential care programs for the ethnic aged. This is particularly relevant with the current trends in health service planning and budget allocations to area-based services.

Specific problems experienced by the aged

Language

The most often reported difficulty experienced by older people of non-English-speaking origin in Australia is the language gap. Table 5.1 shows that over half of the Greek, Italian, Lebanese, Chinese and Vietnamese aged 60 years and older claim that *they speak and understand little English.* This proportion increases with age in all the communities, so that even larger proportions of those aged 70 years and older (those most likely to be in need of health and community support services) are probably unable to communicate in English.

Table 5.1 Aged Persons non-competent* in English Language, by selected Birthplace Groups and Age, Australia 1981

	60-69		70+		Total 60+	
	No.	% of age group	No.	% of age group	No.	% of age group
Baltic states	668	12.1	1278	31.0	1946	20.2
Germany	520	6.0	867	18.0	1387	10.2
Greece	4304	58.8	3533	61.8	7837	60.1
Hungary	654	14.8	932	33.6	1586	22.0
Italy	12 972	52.1	1098	56.1	23 961	53.9
Malta	869	24.0	734	35.7	1603	28.2
Netherlands	375	3.2	537	12.8	912	5.7
Poland	2803	18.8	1900	33.1	4703	22.8
Ukraine	761	26.1	714	55.9	1475	35.1
USSR	1086	28.4	1742	46.8	2828	37.5
Yugoslavia	2815	37.3	2441	54.0	5256	43.5
Egypt	647	20.7	628	39.3	1285	26.9
Lebanon	727	58.7	427	52.8	1154	56.3
China	1972	58.3	1322	65.3	3294	60.9
India	74	1.8	49	1.9	123	1.8
Vietnam	354	86.3	131	87.9	486	89.6
Total non-English-speaking	36 618	28.2	31 769	40.7	68 387	32.9

Source: ABS, 1981 Census, Table 65.
*Census categories 'not well' and 'not at all' were combined.
(ex Australian Institute of Multicultural Affairs, 1985).[12]

While the Lebanese, Chinese and Vietnamese communities have settled in Australia more recently than the European groups, it should be noted that the Australian Institute of Multicultural Affairs[12] found that 91 per cent of the total sample had come to Australia with no English-speaking ability and only 24 per cent reported they had received tuition in English since their arrival. In other words, few English language classes were offered to the early postwar settlers and the great majority would have learned English informally through friends and people at work. Yet in all groups there had been a tendency to learn some English by the age of 40, and to learn more when old.

Often the learned vocabulary, however, would have been work-related and of little use in retirement generally or, more specifically, in discussions of intimate physical and emotional matters.

Lack of English language fluency has widespread implications for the well-being of older migrants. These include:

- social isolation in daily interactions with neighbours, shopkeepers, service providers, acquaintances;
- limited use of mainstream media outlets and therefore limited access to community education on issues relating to growing older, preventive health, current affairs, etc;
- limited knowledge of the Australian social welfare and health services. This is compounded by the fact that many currently ageing migrants come from rural areas or from countries in the early stages of industrialisation; their experiences of ageing in an industrialised society would be quite different from their expectations of growing old in a rural setting.

The Institute found that the ethnic aged experienced greater difficulties in adjusting to retirement than native English speakers. Some of the difficulties related to:

- higher unemployment, less access to part-time work, earlier retirement, fewer working spouses, less well-paid jobs, and a greater unsatisfied desire to work;
- more adjustment problems, a less adequate income, and fewer private sources of income such as lump sum payments, interest or dividends.

Health

The ethnic aged consistently reported poorer health than the Australian-born aged. As a group, aged migrants from English-speaking countries, on all indicators, reported a health status intermediate between the other two groups. The migration experience largely accounts for the difference in health status in old age. The experience has a more negative effect on health when the immigrant has little or no facility with English.

Available data on the use of health programs and services indicate in most cases a lower rate of use across the birthplace groups of the overseas-born. These results appear to reflect differences in the appropriateness of services, rather than differences in health or need of the services.

Social isolation

Older migrants living alone may find it difficult to associate with predominantly English-speaking senior citizen groups or with neighbours and they may have a limited social network within their own ethnic groups. If the ethnic aged live with their families, and their adult children and grandchildren prefer to speak English, they become isolated in their own homes. In fact, one of the most striking findings of the study into the ethnic aged[9] by the Institute of Multicultural Affairs is that the feeling of loneliness among the ethnic aged is not related to living arrangements – a person living alone is not necessarily more desolate than a person living in a large family setting. Colson[9] found that almost half (43 per cent) of the respondents who 'quite often feel lonely' live in a three-generational household, and another quarter (24 per cent) live with their spouse.

Surprising as these results appear at first, once we analyse the content of other questions relating to social relationships (or lack of them), responses cluster on a need to meet contemporaries of similar cultural and linguistic background. For instance, almost half (49.4 per cent) the respondents stated they had no one with whom they could share a common interest or activity. This compares with less than one-fifth of the Anglo-Australian aged (19.5 per cent).

Given that the majority of older migrants live with a spouse or with family members, it appears that respondents look to people outside their immediate family to do things with or to reminisce. Analysis of family composition among older migrants in Australia shows that, if the ethnic aged have a family, it is usually composed of their spouse, adult children, and grandchildren; relatively few have any contemporaries such as cousins, brothers or sisters in Australia. Rowland[14] found that among elderly Australian-born people, 39 per cent had a brother and 51 per cent had a sister living in Sydney, compared with only 11.4 per cent and 18 per cent respectively among the elderly of non-English-speaking origin. The Australian National University survey found, however, that older people draw considerable social, emotional and practical support from extended family members and friends of their own age group.

The ethnic aged who were brought up in one cultural setting but grow old in another may have a great need to validate their current realities with contemporaries of similar cultural background. They may feel a particular need to bridge the often dramatic discontinuities they experienced in their lives, either through war and/or migration to Australia. Children raised in Australia, although they may share some of the values of their parents, nevertheless are not able to empathise with their parents' experience of growing old in Australia. A study by Myerhoff[6] of elderly Jews in Los Angeles found that they felt separated by cultural gaps from their more Americanised children. Research into Mexican and Polish Americans[6] found similar results. These studies also found that individual identification with respective ethnic groups represented a significant resource in dealing with the problems of ageing. The resource consisted of shared symbols and rituals which could be validated with others from similar backgrounds. Such exchange appears to provide meaning and support in old age.

The emphasis on the role of significant peers in older people's lives does not deny the important role of family members in the lives of the ethnic aged. Families often provide primary care, shelter and companionship, but the prevalence of desolation among the ethnic aged in Australia, regardless of whether they live with families or alone, may well point to the lack of opportunities to meet contemporaries of similar ethnic origin.

Family support

The Institute of Multicultural Affairs said in 1983:

> The view is frequently expressed by these service providers that the ethnic aged do not utilise these services because they are cared for by their families, whether co-resident or living in the next suburb, or by their extended families. Consequently, they do not have a need for these services. . .[8]

In fact, there is a tendency among Southern European (and Asian) communities for ageing parents to live with their sons or daughters (see Table 5.2). These estimates clearly indicate that the older the grandparents

Table 5.2 Australia: Percentage of Older Persons in major Birthplace Groups living in three-generational Households

Age group	Birthplace			
	Australia	UK/Eire	North Europe	South Europe
	%	%	%	%
60-64	1.9	2.1	3.5	3.8
65-69	2.6	4.1	3.9	6.3
70-74	4.0	4.7	6.6	21.4
75 +	7.5	11.5	12.5	32.2

(Source: ABS 1981 Census, one per cent sample of households). ex: National Research Institute of Gerontology and Geriatric Services. Occasional Paper No. 6. The Ageing of Ethnic Populations in Australia, 1984.

are, the more likely it is that they will move into the household of their children. These tendencies are more pronounced among the Southern Europeans than in the Northern European groups. British and Australian-born are least likely to live in a three-generational household.

Brewer,[15] conducting a study with older Greek- and Italian-born migrants in Victoria, suggests that it is not known for certain if the greater likelihood of Southern Europeans living in a family setting emanates from choice or the lack of alternative options. Brewer quotes Rowland[14] who concludes that 'high probabilities of living with relatives are associated with recency of residential movement, non-English-speaking background, low socio-economic status and larger number of children'. MSJ Keys Young,[16] studying the more recently arrived older migrants who entered Australia under the Family Reunion scheme, came to similar conclusions.

The Australian Institute of Multicultural Affairs[8] comments that, in all the ethnic groups it surveyed, living with the family is not typical as long as one's spouse is alive. However, once one of the couple dies, the other is more likely to move in with their children. Of the ethnic aged who do not have a spouse, the Institute found that 38 per cent live alone and 61 per cent live with family members or other persons. This compares with 60 per cent of Australian-born who live alone. Table 5.3 shows the proportions of persons living alone in different groups.

Table 5.3 Australia: Percentage of Older Persons living Alone

Age group	Australia	UK/Eire	Northern Europe	Southern Europe
	%	%	%	%
60-64	15.7	15.2	17.3	5.1
65-69	21.9	17.9	20.7	12.7
70-74	29.1	26.6	27.2	15.6
75+	33.2	27.1	29.9	13.6

(Source: ABS 1981 Census, one per cent sample of individuals). ex: National Research Institute of Gerontology and Geriatric Services. Occasional Paper No. 6. The Ageing of Ethnic Populations in Australia, 1984.

It should be noted that significant proportions of married British, Australian and North-Eastern European women now in the 60-plus age group have never had children – 17.9 per cent; 12.4 per cent; 17.7 per cent respectively – compared with less than 4 per cent of Southern European women. In other words, fewer of the Anglo- and North-Eastern Europeans have the choice of moving in with their children when they can no longer cope.

It is also important to note that, due to postwar immigration patterns, there are more older males than females in the Northern and Eastern European communities, as well as in the Italian and Maltese communities. For a variety of reasons these men may never have formed a family and, because they have often worked in isolated country areas (e.g. on the Snowy Mountain Scheme or in remote mining fields), they are likely to have a limited social network in old age and so experience considerable social isolation. And because most of the generalist recreational programs are geared to native-English-speaking females, older single males may find few recreational activities they would feel attracted to join.

Some research has been initiated in Australia into the problems experienced by families who care for an aged person at home (Social Welfare Research Centre).[17,18] The Australian Institute of Multicultural Affairs[9] considers the share of aged care provided by the immediate family is significantly higher among those of non-English-speaking background than among other migrants or the Australian-born. The inequality of care responsibilities falling on a few individuals, rather than on the broader community, applies with greater force among most immigrant groups.

Considering the significant role that ethnic families assume in the care of the frail aged, and the current policy direction of developing community services to prevent early institutional care, it is crucial that the ethnic aged and their carers are consulted to establish the particular difficulties they may experience in gaining access to existing community support services. Also, variations between groups as to the perceived appropriateness of these services need to be considered.

The Institute summarises: Access to community services is severely restricted among the ethnic aged. While all the needy aged in the community face a massive shortfall in services, the problems are especially acute for the ethnic aged. Few know about community services and the level of use is low. Even when services are available, they are of limited value in alleviating many of the difficulties experienced by the ethnic aged: virtually no assistance is available for shopping or in moving around in the community and language/cultural barriers further limit use of community services such as Meals-on-Wheels and homekeeping services.

Making use of services

Studies have shown that the ethnic aged are just as likely as native English-speakers to use the services of the general practitioner.[7,16,19] When bilingual doctors[20] were consulted about the particular difficulties the ethnic aged experienced in making use of specific services, several commented that patients felt insecure, or confused about the health care system, and needed reassurance or clarification of diagnosis, the purpose of the proposed treatment, or related questions. There may also be a reluctance to accept strangers into their homes, all of which contribute to the extra load on the carer family. Yet, generally, doctors considered that once the purpose of the services was fully explained to the ethnic aged, they readily accepted them (e.g. rehabilitation services, aids for the disabled, and paramedical services).

Accommodation

Brewer[15] comments on Australia's housing stock which is usually unsuitable for large families. The Australian Council on the Ageing and the Department of Social Security[21] found that overcrowding was highest for those from Southern Europe and non-English-speaking countries outside Europe. Little wonder, then, that intergenerational conflict is reputedly high. Yet, Brewer found, if asked their preference for care once the aged could no longer cope, the first choice of the majority was family care; few of the ethnic aged would contemplate nursing home care. In fact, the Australian Institute of Multicultural Affairs[9] estimated in 1985 that, of those aged 75 years and over, 9 per cent of the Australian-born were nursing home patients compared with only 5 per cent of those from non-English-speaking countries in the same age group. Furthermore, only an estimated 3 per cent of hostel residents were of non-English-speaking background. In other words, institutional care was seen as a last resort among the ethnic aged.

Unfamiliarity with the concept of nursing home care, a cultural belief in caring for members of the family, and fear of social isolation of the ethnic aged in English-speaking nursing homes would be the main pressures on the family to care for the aged at home.

Nursing home care

While there are a few ethno-specific nursing homes in New South Wales (e.g. the Chinese, Greek, Hungarian, Italian, Jewish and Russian communities have developed or acquired a nursing home), about 80 per cent of ethnic patients are estimated to be in English-speaking nursing homes.[9,11] Two brief surveys conducted by the NSW Council on the Ageing[20,22] found that the ethnic aged in a generalist nursing home were most likely to have no one with whom they could communicate in their first language, since there are few nursing homes where there are two or more patients of the same ethnic origin. The tendency to prefer the native language, together with the increasing difficulty of speaking English when frail, contribute greatly to the social isolation experienced by the ethnic aged in predominantly English-speaking institutions.[23] There being only one, or possibly two, patients of similar ethnic background would also make it difficult for the management to make allowances for cultural differences in terms of food, recreation and religious observances.[20,24]

Given the projected rapid increase among those aged 75 years and over in specific ethnic communities over the next two decades, the Australian Institute of Multicultural Affairs[12] concludes:

> To give greater attention to ethnic and cultural factors in the running of general nursing homes and hostels would require some adaptation of existing service provision, including a re-appraisal of recruiting strategies and staff training. It also seems necessary to develop and test new approaches, such as the bringing together of residents by birthplace, ethnicity, cultural or language background. This could be done, for example, by accommodating together people from similar backgrounds in a single ward or wing, employing a co-ordinator with the appropriate background and qualifications to oversee the day-to-day operation of such a ward, and establishing and maintaining close links with ethnic communities from which the residents are drawn. This would be particularly feasible in large institutions, and may also be possible for institutions in close proximity.
>
> At the same time, there remains a valid case for maintaining and continuing to support the development of ethno-specific accommodation to cater for the ethnic aged, who clearly prefer to live in such facilities, which generally operate in close contact with the relevant ethnic community. For services with particular clienteles to be funded by government under general programs is not unusual in the Australian context, nor is it a case of privileged treatment.

Demographic changes taking place among many birthplace groups clearly indicate an inevitable demand for increasing provision of accommodation. This is most likely to be the case for the Dutch, Polish and Yugoslav communities, where the number of those aged 75 years and over will increase more than five-fold in the period 1981-2001. Less dramatic increases, but all more than trebling, will occur among the Maltese, German, Greek, Italian, Russian, Ukrainian and Hungarian communities.

Possible solutions to problems identified

The ageing of ethnic communities in Australia coincides with changes in the overall policy direction of limiting the growth of nursing home care and further expansion of community/hostel care – as described in the *Nursing Homes and Hostels Review.*[26]

Upon completion of the ethnic aged research project by the Institute of Multicultural Affairs, an interdepartmental working party was formed to respond to the implications of the finding.[25]

Institutional care services

Both reports have developed recommendations for more appropriate services for the increasingly pluralist aged population. For example, while there are relatively few ethno-specific nursing homes, for a variety of reasons, the smaller ethnic groups are in no position to acquire or run a nursing home.

Thus, the *Nursing Homes and Hostels Review*[26] recommends that current capital funding arrangements under the Aged or Disabled Persons Homes Act should be made more flexible, to allow for 100 per cent government funding to ethnic groups who cannot afford to raise their share of the capital cost but who warrant special consideration in nursing care (Recommendation 18).

Another way to use existing generalist nursing homes more effectively would be to diversify their services provision to match the needs of specific community groups. There has been little planning, for instance, in the placement of individuals of specific linguistic/cultural origin into nursing homes. Past attempts to group ethnic patients of similar cultural or linguistic origin in designated generalist homes have failed. This is partly because of *ad hoc* placement procedures from acute hospitals to the next available nursing home bed, partly the reportedly long waiting periods to gain access to particular nursing homes.

The introduction of area-based multidisciplinary assessment teams may facilitate the placement of patients of similar cultural/linguistic background into designated nursing homes to allow for the development of such clusters.

Another difficulty in catering for the specific needs of a group of ethnic patients in generalist nursing homes is that a great proportion of such homes are private, profit-making establishments. They are run on tight budgets, and rely on efficient management with expertise in the bulk-buying of foodstuffs. Nursing care is delivered with the minimum number of staff needed to provide a standard of care compliant with the hygienic and physical requirements laid down by state governments.

The *Nursing Homes and Hostels Review* acknowledges some of these difficulties and recommends the development of 'innovative project programs'. Ways should be explored whereby the management of private and non-profit nursing homes could apply for recurrent funding to allow them to cater for a (small) number of non-English-speaking patients of similar cultural/linguistic origin. This could mean a willingness to provide ethno-specific food styles; a policy of hiring bilingual staff of a particular language background; developing culturally and linguistically appropriate recreational activities; encouraging networks with relevant ethnic community members; fostering links with suitable bilingual doctors; and financing the holding of beds (when required) to allow the transfer or placement of ethnic patients into these designated homes.[20]

The Ethnic Aged Working Party[25] also recommends funds to enable a number of nursing homes with five or more residents of a particular language group to employ bilingual ethnic aides, on a flexible basis, to help in the development and implementation of care programs. Preference should be given to facilities where there is a lack of professional staff proficient in the language of residents (Recommendation 19).

More generally, the task force recommends that the Commonwealth/State Working party on Standards in Nursing Homes ensure that the standards currently being developed for nursing homes include requirements that the care and lifestyle provided should reflect the cultural and religious backgrounds of residents (Recommendation 21).

Community support services

There are many services of potential use to the ethnic aged living in the community and it is difficult to generalise because of this diversity. The programs have different aims and are under different auspices, and there is also considerable variation within each program.

Nevertheless, the Ethnic Aged Working Party[25] recommends that the Department of Community Services negotiate with State/Territory government departments responsible for the day-to-day administration of Home and Community Care Programs (HACC) to seek their agreement that:

- work be undertaken to target high-need ethnic communities and to identify service providers to develop specific proposals ensuring delivery of services to these communities:
- contract/funding agreements between service providers and the State/Territory governments impose a responsibility to ensure access to the services by ethnic communities, in consultation with ethnic organisations (Recommendation 5).

In particular, the Ethnic Aged Working Party has recognised that the networks, experience and skills of ethnic community agencies would be invaluable in addressing these needs.

The involvement of ethnic organisations in the welfare of the aged cannot be overemphasised. These organisations may act in an advisory capacity to government, be involved in the planning of service provision and, in line with current policy direction to 'mainstream public services', provide complementary services to community members as is customary with other voluntary sector agencies.

Most medium to large ethnic communities organise regular group meetings on a regional or local level to enable older members to go on joint outings, learn about support services, or simply enjoy one another's company. Smaller community groups tend to meet less frequently. Brewer[15] reports that the great majority of ethnic aged in the Victorian project said they would welcome assistance outside their families in developing social outlets. Guthrie[12] explored the needs of older Italians and concluded that what they need most is the opportunity to reflect on old times and quiet conversations with contemporaries. This could be fairly easily organised on a local level.

More thought needs to be given to developing meaningful and culturally appropriate activities for older men. Past experience, however, shows that such community development occurs only when bilingual catalyst workers are employed and mainstream organisations co-operate by providing meeting places and transport facilities. Above all, it must be accepted that the ethnic aged feel most comfortable in the company of their own cultural/language group. This does not mean that they do not wish to meet fellow pensioners of different cultural or linguistic background, including English speakers. Exchange of views across cultural groups can make lives richer and more active and foster a greater mutual understanding. But, given the language gap among the aged, it must be recognised that it may be strenuous – both for native English speakers to listen to potentially broken English and for second language speakers to make themselves understood in English.

There is also scope for further development of English language maintenance classes,[12,15] particularly for those who have been retrenched from the workforce before they reached retirement age and who in previous years may never have had the opportunity to attend English language classes. They often feel bored and useless and need new challenges to develop some of their skills.

One of the greatest difficulties faced by ethnic welfare organisations is reaching out to isolated members who have lost contact with their own ethnic group but find it difficult to link up with mainstream society.[24] Community nurses, welfare workers and doctors in contact with isolated individuals can help by encouraging them to join local activity or social groups. To be able to do this, they need accurate information about when and where ethnic groups meet. Thus, more detailed information about mainstream and ethno-specific services must be made available so that referers can put individuals in touch with suitable social/recreational groups and support services. Today's computer facilities within hospital or local government services should enable maintenance of up-to-date information on local services, which can be made available to those in direct contact with the aged.

For example, the Service Directory for the Aged, Inner Western Suburbs,[20] lists:

- services provided in the home;
- assessment and rehabilitation services;
- social groups, including those where languages other than English predominate;
- ethno-specific clinical services.

The advantages of having the aged involved in the family need to be stressed. We can learn from the extended family arrangements that sometimes characterise the older migrant's family. Instead of discarding the values and experiences of older members, their families can be enriched by incorporating these into their daily life. Although it is not often reported, the aged can contribute much to the family's well-being.

In the planning, resource allocation and diversification of existing mainstream services, or the development of ethno-specific services, it is crucial to recognise that ethnic communities are geographically widely scattered. This means that on a subregional or area level there is a multiplicity of languages spoken which makes it very complex to diversify the services to specific community needs. There must be cross-area or regional planning, particularly under the program funding proposals, as there may be insufficient numbers of a particular ethnic group at a local level to justify efforts to reach out to them with a specific program. These issues need to be thoroughly discussed and recommendations developed as to how we can most effectively diversify mainstream services to meet the needs of the multilingual/multicultural ageing population in an equitable manner.

Nursing roles in relation to the aged migrant

Clearly it is impossible to be completely familiar with all the attitudes and practices of all the ethnic groups with whom the nurse has contact. What is needed is the development of a broad awareness of the behaviour of different migrant groups and a willingness to respond to patients and help them in terms of their own values. These may vary, depending on past experience of health services in the country of origin. Older migrants may come from rural areas, cities, developing countries or technologically advanced Western countries, where their experience of nursing may be very different. Paramedical professions, such as occupational or physiotherapists, may be unknown to them and they will probably have a different attitude to nurses, hospitals and nursing home services.

Cultural sensitivity

Nurses need to develop a sensitivity to the significance of cultural factors in their own and other people's lives, as these elements pervade all we think, do and say. This cultural awareness can be developed by studying different groups through reading and attending courses, and by using everyday opportunities to watch, listen attentively and talk to patients and their families. If patients' cultural values can be identified, and they can be nursed within that context, then communication will be greatly enhanced. Where family members exist, their role is to show concern and affection. Not to visit a person in hospital, for example, would be considered disrespectful in some of the European, Middle Eastern and Asian communities.[27]

In European and Asian societies the aged are usually well respected. In their own language they would be addressed in the formal mode and by their surname. Changing to the more intimate and informal way of address, using the first name, should be negotiated between individuals and the initiative to do so left to the older person. Elderly ethnic people in Australian institutions may take offence when called by their first name by a much younger person.[28]

The nurse's feelings

It is important for nurses to recognise their own feelings when working with the migrant aged. Initially, feelings of inadequacy, frustration and anger may be experienced as the older migrant fails to respond in the way one's culture and professional training have conditioned expectations. Differences in cultural modes of expression may include:

- reactions to illness in general
- reactions to pain
- responses to approaching death
- family responses to illness and death.

With today's increasing emphasis on the right of the individual to have access to information concerning him has come a more open approach to the discussion of death. It is now quite customary in Australia to insist on telling patients that they are going to die, but this practice upsets most people of a non-English-speaking cultural background. In most ethnic communities it is considered that a dying person does not need to be told; they know that death is near, though they may deny it or not speak about it at all. Some ethnic community members may consider it cruel to tell the patient of his imminent death. However, the family should be told. Their role is to support the patient by showing affection and respect and by providing emotional comfort. Family members may not necessarily talk about death to the patient, even if they know that he or she knows . . . they try to make the patient as happy as possible.[27]

If these cultural differences are identified and talked about with others, for example, at staff conferences or the handover of the nursing report, then a major block will be removed and communication will flow more easily. Also, nursing care plans should include ethnic considerations.

Communication

The importance of congruent non-verbal communication with what is spoken cannot be too highly stressed; the aged migrant often comes from a culture where feelings and emotions are more highly valued and understood than they are in our own, and any differences between what the nurse says and does will be quickly spotted.

When talking to the aged migrant who speaks some English, take care to speak slowly and clearly. Try to avoid the use of slang, colloquialisms and abstract terms. Choose short, simple sentences and words in everyday use, and speak at a normal volume. Unless the patient has a hearing impairment, raising the voice will not help him to understand a foreign language. The aged migrant will feel more secure with the nurse who states clearly what she is aiming to do, and what her expectations are. Otherwise, confusion, fear and suspicion will result and lead to a lack of co-operation.

Interpreters who are specially trained to work in the health field should be used wherever possible by the nurse. They will be invaluable in important areas of prevention, such as cancer detection, mental health, bereavement and rehabilitation. Their use is particularly important during the nursing assessment and the treatment plan, both for the client and the health professional. A clear understanding of what is to happen will facilitate treatment and rehabilitation. Generally speaking, it is unwise to use domestic staff or family members as interpreters. This is a situation which often arises, but it can result in problems rather than therapeutic help. The patient may be embarrassed, for example, or withhold personal information.

Resources

Videos and films are available which portray issues affecting migrants and help to promote sensitivity and an understanding of cultural differences. These can be obtained from migrant organisations, colleges and universities, and health departments. Information centres and other organisations provide practical assistance to aged migrants and their families.

For details, consult the latest (1987) edition of the *Directory of Ethnic Community Organisations in Australia*, produced by the Department of Immigration and Ethnic Affairs and published by the Australian Government Publishing Service, Canberra. Other useful addresses are listed below. The following organisations may be used as initial contacts to locate further specific resources.

1. Federation of Ethnic Communities' Councils of Australia, 541 George Street, Sydney 2000. (This is the national umbrella organisation of ethnic communities and deals mainly with national issues.)
2. Department of Immigration and Ethnic Affairs, Canberra. (This Federal department has regional offices in all States and may be contacted for information on bilingual service providers and other resources.)
3. Ethnic Communities Council. (This body exists in each State and the address can be found in the telephone book.)
4. Ethnic Affairs Commission. (This State body is usually part of the Premier's Department; the address can be found in the State Government section of the telephone book.)
5. Various State Government health and welfare services exist (such as the Department of Youth and Community Services in New South Wales); again their addresses can be found at the front of the telephone book. Their libraries contain information on translated material, research on ethnic groups, and catalogues of films and videos in other languages.

Questions

1. Why has there been so little interest in the aged of non-English-speaking origin?
2. Describe the position of the aged migrant in his own culture.
3. What problems are created by migration for:
   (a) older people, and

(b) their children and grandchildren?

4. What can be done for the aged of non-English-speaking origin generally?
5. Discuss the role of the nurse in relation to the ethnic aged.

Task

1. Develop a demographic profile of the various cultural groups in your local government area.
2. Evaluate the extent to which the needs of one of the groups identified in 1 above are currently being met by health and other community services.
3. Where deficiencies are identified in 2, describe how these could be remedied.

References

1. Morrisey MJ. Some considerations on provision of welfare services to migrants. In Jamrozik A. Provision of welfare services to immigrants. Paper presented at EWRC seminar, University of NSW, 1986.
2. Australian Council on Population and Ethnic Affairs. Multiculturalism for all Australians. Canberra: AGPS, 1982.
3. Forum 'Changing Times, Changing Needs'. Greek Welfare Centre, COASIT (Italian Association of Assistance, Sydney), Yugoslav Australian Association Information and Welfare Centre, 1986.
4. National Population Council. Access and Equity. Canberra: AGPS, 1982.
5. Crandall RC. Gerontology: a behavioural science approach. Massachusetts: Addison-Wesley Publishing Co. 1980.
6. Bengtson VL. Ethnicity and ageing: problems and issues in current social inquiry. In Gelfund DE, Kutzik AJ, eds. Ethnicity and aging: theory, research and policy. New York: Springer, 1979.
7. Kendig HL, Gibson D, Rowland DR, Hemer JM. Health, welfare and family in later life. Canberra: Australian National University, Research School of Social Sciences, 1983.
8. Australian Institute of Multicultural Affairs. Papers on the ethnic aged. Melbourne, 1983.
9. Australian Institute of Multicultural Affairs. Community and institutional care for aged migrants in Australia – research findings. Melbourne, 1986.
10. Australian Bureau of Statistics. Census of population and housing. Canberra: ABS, 1986.
11. Australian Bureau of Statistics. Census of population and housing. Canberra: ABS, 1981.

12. Australian Institute of Multicultural Affairs. Ageing in a multicultural society: the situation of migrants from non-English speaking countries. Melbourne: AIMA, 1985.
13. Polish Welfare and Information Bureau. Ageing in Australia: Polish aged needs and services. Sydney: PWIB, 1984.
14. Rowland DT. The family circumstances of the ethnic aged. In Papers on the Ethnic Aged. Melbourne, Australia: Institute of Multicultural Affairs, 1983.
15. Brewer G. Ethnic aged and local government. A study of the needs of Italian and Greek aged residents in the municipalities of Northcote and Brunswick. Federal Department of Local Government and Administrative Services, Victoria, 1985.
16. MSJ Keys Young Planners. Family reunion study. Prepared for the Department of Immigration and Ethnic Affairs, 1984.
17. Kinnear D, Graycar D. Family care of elderly people: Australian perspective. University of NSW, Social Welfare Centre: Report No.23, 1982.
18. Rossiter C, Kinnear D, Graycar D. Family care of elderly people: 1983 Survey results. University of NSW Social Welfare Centre: Report No.38, 1984.
19. Shaw D, Bryson L. Social support network in an urban community. Melbourne, Australia: Institute of Family Studies, 1984.
20. Schappi, U. Ethnic Aged Project: a report on diversifying community support and residential service delivery to meet the needs of elderly people of non-English-speaking background. Migrant Health Services Unit, Southern Metropolitan Health Region, Area Geriatric Services, Royal Prince Alfred Hospital and Area Health Service, NSW Dept of Health, 1987.
21. Australian Council on the Ageing. Older people at home. A final survey report. Canberra: ACA, 1985.
22. New South Wales Council on the Ageing. A directory of services for non-English speaking patients in NSW hostels and nursing homes. Sydney: NSW Council on the Ageing, 1984.
23. Moriatis S. The migrant aged. In Howe AL, ed. Towards an older Australia. Queensland, Australia: University of Queensland Press, 1981.
24. Schappi U. Options for migrant communities. Australian Journal on Ageing 1983; 2: 1.
25. Department of Community Services. Strategies for change. Report of the Ethnic Aged Working Party, Canberra: Department of Community Services, 1986.
26. Department of Community Services. Nursing homes and hostels review. Canberra: AGPS, 1986.
27. Migrant Health Unit. Cultural diversity and health care: a guide for health professionals. Sydney: Health Commission of New South Wales, 1981.
28. Phillip Institute of Technology. The immigrant patient in an Australian nursing home. Victoria: School of Community Studies, 1985.

Further reading

Bottomley G, de Lepervanche M. Ethnicity, class and gender in Australia. Sydney: Allen & Unwin, 1984.

Brink JP. Transcultural nursing. Englewood Cliffs: Prentice-Hall, 1976.

Leininger M. Care, the essence of nursing and health. Slack Inco, 1984.

Leininger M. Nursing and anthropology: two worlds to blend. New York: John Wiley and Sons, 1970.

Leininger M. Transcultural nursing. New York: Masson, 1979.

Martin J. The ethnic dimension. Sydney: Allen & Unwin, 1981.

Storer D, ed. Ethnic family values in Australia. Compiled by the Institute of Family Studies. Australia: Prentice Hall, 1985.

Chapter 6

Health Assessment of the Older Person

Objectives

To enable the reader to:

1. identify and describe briefly the five-step model of the Nursing Process as proposed by Bloch;
2. list the reasons why the assessment of older patients may be somewhat different from that of younger ones and describe the possible adjustments for this that the nurse can make;
3. appreciate that a knowledge of the normal ageing process and altered patterns of disease in old age is important when assessing the older person;
4. identify and describe the three techniques in the assessment process;
5. specify some examples of physical assessment skills the nurse should master;
6. appreciate the importance of recording assessment findings;
7. have an understanding of the information that could be obtained by using a standard nursing assessment form;
8. describe briefly what is meant by Nursing Diagnosis.

Various attempts have been made in recent years to define the nature of nursing. For the purposes of this chapter I have chosen a definition which captures this quite simply:

> The purpose of nursing is to directly or indirectly supply the help a patient or client requires to meet his need.[1]

The nursing process

If this definition is accepted, then it may be said that the goal identified is best accomplished through the Nursing Process. This can be applied in any nursing situation and allows the collection of data which provides the nurse with a comprehensive view of the patient or client. Some writers[2-7] have identified four steps in the nursing process:

- Assessment
- Planning
- Implementation
- Evaluation

I prefer to use the five-step model proposed by Bloch[8] which delineates 'definition of the problem' as a clearly recognisable step in the process. We now have:

1. Collection of data
2. Definition of the problem
3. Planning of the intervention
4. Implementation of the intervention
5. Evaluation of the intervention

Collection of data. This involves the nurse in gathering objective and subjective data about the physical, social and emotional aspects of the health status of the individual.

Definition of the problem. Here the nurse makes decisions about the patient's problem/s, strengths, limitations and methods of adapting to the problem/s. The nurse formulates a clear statement of the clinical nursing problems which she has to manage, e.g. depression related to realisation of inability to remember events and places. This statement, or nursing diagnosis, also suggests the necessary intervention required, e.g. the patient will need constant reality orientation by nursing staff.

Planning the intervention. Here the nurse decides on appropriate actions to solve the defined problem/s.

Implementing the intervention involves carrying out the planned nursing actions.

Evaluating the intervention. In this final step the nurse determines the degree of effectiveness of the action/s taken in solving the problem/s defined.

The advantages of the nursing process have been well documented. McCarthy,[7] for example, notes the following:

- It gives individualised care, especially as it advocates nurse to patient allocation;
- It offers a framework for teaching the theory behind the physical nursing skills;
- It makes the best use of resources by setting priorities;
- It increases job satisfaction by making it easier for the nurse's individual contribution to be recognised.

To these I must add one of its most important advantages: it contributes to more efficient and effective nursing care, thus producing positive benefits for the patient/client.

Assessing the older patient

The information collected by the nurse through assessment of the older adult will provide a comprehensive view of his physiological and psychosocial status. Preferably, assessment should occur at every interaction with the patient, as the status of many older adults may fluctuate rapidly.

It is important for the nurse to realise that the assessment process will be somewhat different from that adopted with younger patients.[9,10] Reasons for this may include:

- decreased vision
- decreased hearing
- memory loss
- depression
- chronic illness
- feelings of diminished control
- the aged may tell their story more slowly
- the aged may tire more easily
- the aged will have longer histories[11,12]

The assessing nurse will need to be alert to these and other problems and make the necessary adjustments by:

- taking extra time with the older person;
- coming back several times to obtain a complete history;
- being aware of the comfort of the elderly patient during the interview.[9,10,12]

Generally, the nurse should:

- collect pertinent information (e.g. to what extent will a detailed history of pregnancies be helpful?);

- ascertain how the older person evaluates and views his total health picture and the problem/s being experienced;
- ask the older person to describe a typical 24-hour period;
- remember that the older person may not always recollect information about earlier illnesses, operations, etc;
- be aware of her own feelings about old age and older people;
- talk to the older person's relatives, friends, neighbours and general practitioner to fill out the picture gained through history taking;
- be sure to arrange for an assessment of the older person's activities of daily living (ADL) to be done in their own home;
- possess a good knowledge of the effects of the normal ageing process on the older adult (see Chapter 2);
- clearly recognise the altered pattern of disease in old age (see Chapter 8).[9-11,13]

Methods of assessment

Techniques used in the assessment process include the interview, observation and a physical examination.

The interview

Basically, an interview is a conversation between two or more people which is purposeful and serious.[14] Interviews may be structured or unstructured. The nursing interview will include structured questions but should not be so inflexible that the interviewing nurse cannot follow important cues provided by the older client.

The nursing interview will help the nurse to gather vital information about the older patient, which will then enable her to provide appropriate nursing care. It will also help to form a relationship with the older person that will help him to trust and confide in the interviewing nurse. Finally, the nurse in this situation may learn something about herself and her way of relating to others.[15,16]

No nursing history will ever be complete, but with practice, guidance and self-awareness the nurse can learn to talk with the older adult and obtain a comprehensive, organised set of data. To do that, it is necessary to know what information is required, how to get it, and how to build a relationship as the interview proceeds.[14]

It helps to set the stage for the interview by obtaining identifying data early in the interview. This will include the older person's age, sex, marital status, address, occupation and religion. This information will provide useful insights into his life experiences and give an appreciation of the individuality of the older patient.[5-7]

Ideally, the environment for the interview should be quiet and private, although this may be difficult on a busy ward. The nurse and older patient should sit in clear view of each other, preferably at eye level. Ventilation and lighting are also important issues. The placement of the nurse's chair in relation to the patient should be thought about before the interview.[14]

When greeting older patients it is important to be aware of how they like to be addressed – Mr, Mrs, Miss or by some other title. The nurse should introduce herself by name and explain clearly her relationship to the patient's care.[4]

The nurse must be alert to the patient's comfort during the interview. It is helpful to ask how the patient is feeling and to watch for any signs of discomfort.[9,10]

Opening questions will aim to find out why the older person is in hospital or has come seeking help. Questions of a general nature may encourage a freer response. As the older person answers specific questions and responds generally the nurse can pick up cues provided and follow these.

As the interview proceeds, the nurse should be careful not to ask double questions as these may be particularly confusing to the older adult. Deal with one point at a time. The 'why' question may not be particularly helpful as often the client may not know the reason why. Open-ended questions such as: 'what do you enjoy doing most?' are often more helpful than questions which can be answered by a yes or no. It is important, of course, for the nurse to listen carefully at all times to the older person's answers.[14-16]

Many illnesses in old age have complex psychosocial and pathophysiological causes,[18-20] and patients often have complicated feelings about themselves, their illnesses and treatment procedures. The nurse will need to listen actively for cues to these worrying aspects. The client can then be guided into telling more about these areas.[9,10] Some specific interviewing techniques that the nurse may use to help this occur include:

- **Facilitation.** Here the nurse by posture, actions and words encourages the patient to say more.
- **Reflection.** Repetition of the older person's words encourages him to give more details. It serves as a mirror in which the interviewee can see his feelings and thoughts reflected.
- **Clarification.** The interviewer will sometimes need to clarify what the older patient has had difficulty in expressing clearly.
- **Empathic responses** include recognition and actions that show understanding and acceptance. Statements such as 'I understand', and gently placing an arm around the patient at an appropriate time are expressions of empathy.[13,14]

After completing the questions it is helpful to conclude the interview in such a way that the older patient understands that the interview is about to end. Sometimes a concluding statement is made. It is also helpful to check that the interviewee has understood what has taken place during the discussion. Finally, it might be helpful to indicate to the older patient when the next interview will take place.[14]

A sample check list of desirable interviewer behaviours is included below. You are encouraged to use this in interview situations and to ask a colleague to assess your interviews in terms of the check list.

Desirable Interviewer Behaviours

1. **Initial contact**
   Greeting
   Welcoming smile
   Introduction
   Invitation to sit
2. **Attending**
   Positioning
   Posture
   Looking
   Responding
3. **Listening**
   Accurate reflection of feelings
   Accurate reflection of content
   Handling of pauses
   Understanding non-verbal behaviour
   Use of open-ended questions
4. **Constructive action**
   Identification of alternatives and their consequence
   Client choice of best alternative
   Plan of action
   Conclusion of interview

Interviewer attitudes
Warmth
Empathy
Genuineness

Achievement of helping goals
Client self-exploration
Client self-understanding
Client-initiated constructive action

Interviewer's self-assessment
Did you recognise errors in any of the above points?

Comments

(Reproduced with permission of School of Nursing, Cumberland College of Health Sciences)

Observation

In this technique of assessment the nurse uses all the senses to gather useful information about how the older adult is functioning physically and psychosocially. Behaviour to be observed might include the following:

- mental status
- physical traits
- sleeping habits
- reactions to medications
- speech
- appetite/nutritional status
- mobility
- personal hygiene
- bowel and bladder function
- mood
- attitudes
- posture

Physical examination

Nurses need to be able to assess health through physical examination, especially in the nursing home and community setting where access to a doctor may be somewhat limited. Physical examination will provide information beneficial to early recognition of problems and thus ensure prompt treatment or referral.[9-11]

The following are examples of specific physical assessment skills that the nurse should master.*

Cardiovascular system

1. Anatomical landmarks
   (a) identify the ribs and the interspaces on the anterior chest wall;
   (b) surface mark the borders of the heart on the anterior chest wall and know the approximate anatomical location of the chambers of the heart.
2. Arterial pulses
   (a) locate the pulses – radial, brachial, carotid, femoral, popliteal, posterior tibial, and dorsalis pedis;
   (b) make the following observations on an arterial pulse: rate, rhythm, character, volume, condition of the vessel wall;
   (c) measure the blood pressure accurately using a sphygmomanometer.
3. The praecordium
   (a) locate the apex beat and assess the character of the cardial impulse.
4. Percussion
   (a) define the right and left borders of the heart.
5. Auscultation
   (a) locate the four auscultatory areas (mitral, tricuspid, aortic, pulmonary) on the praecordium;
   (b) identify the first and second sound in each area, thereby defining the diastolic and systolic intervals.
6. Peripheral vascular system
   (a) recognise the signs of impaired blood supply to a limb;
   (b) recognise the signs and symptoms of venous thrombosis in a limb.

Respiratory system

1. Locate:
   (a) the sternal angle;
   (b) second rib;
   (c) intercostal spaces;
   (d) third thoracic spine posteriorly;
   (e) lower border of the right and left lungs;
   (f) interlobar groove (sulcus).

---

*Source: School of Nursing, Cumberland College of Health Sciences: Associate Diploma in Clinical Nursing Studies (Gerontological Nursing).

2. Palpate:
   (a) cardiac impulse (apex beat);
   (b) trachea;
   (c) equality of respiratory movements;
   (d) elicit vocal fremitus and compare one side of the lung with the other.
3. Percussion
   (a) demonstrate the correct percussion technique;
   (b) percuss out the lower borders of the lungs;
   (c) appreciate the changes in percussion note associated with underlying conditions in the lung.
4. Auscultation
   (a) differentiate vesicular from bronchial breathing;
   (b) appreciate conditions which alter breathing sounds;
   (c) recognise added sounds (ronchi and rales).

Abdomen

1. Identify the regions of the abdomen.
2. Demonstrate the correct technique for general palpation of the abdomen.
3. Demonstrate the correct technique for palpating the following – liver, spleen, urinary bladder, right and left kidneys.
4. Recall the features to be looked for if an intra-abdominal swelling is palpable.
5. Demonstrate how the presence of ascites may be detected.
6. By percussion demonstrate whether an intra-abdominal structure is solid (fluid-filled) or hollow.
7. Demonstrate the lower border of the liver by percussion.
8. Recognise normal bowel sounds.
9. Identify the sites of occurrence of common hernias and be able to test for the presence of a hernia.

Eyes

1. Demonstrate the ability to assess visual acuity using appropriate procedures including Snellen's test chart.
2. Demonstrate the confrontation method of assessing the visual fields.
3. Be able to draw the visual pathways from the retinae to the cortex and state the visual field defect produced by damage to (a) an optic nerve; (b) an optic tract; and (c) the occipital cortex of one hemisphere.
4. Test for the presence of the light reflex (direct and consensual), accommodation reflex and corneal reflex.

5. Test for the actions of the extra-ocular muscles.
6. Assess ocular tension clinically.
7. Demonstrate the correct technique for using an ophthalmoscope.

Ears

1. Demonstrate the correct technique of examination of the external ear using an electric auriscope.
2. Recall the appearance of the normal tympanic membrane.
3. Demonstrate the simple clinical tests for hearing loss (ticking of watch, whispered voice, etc).
4. Be able to perform and interpret the tuning fork tests (Weber's and Rinne's).
5. Describe the principle of the caloric test.

Network assessment

A fourth method of patient assessment is to be aware of the network of people to which the patient belongs. Network assessment helps to promote the physical and emotional well-being of clients and their families through early identification of problems and appropriate intervention.

The assessing nurse must obtain an understanding of the characteristics and dynamics of networks and their meaning to the older person. This information will help formulate questions at the time of the interview. The knowledge gained will help all those involved to plan and implement services to meet the client's needs.

Cole[20] has identified ten aspects of the older person's social network that would be of interest:

- size of the network;
- degree of variety in the types of people making up the network;
- its spatial distribution;
- the degree of interconnection between members;
- the degree to which the network revolves around one particular person;
- the basis of the relationship (kinship versus ritual);
- duration and frequency of contact;
- resources exchanged in the relationship;
- the directions in which transactions flow;
- the intensity and variety of types of interactions.

Ewing[21] proposes that interaction patterns – communication skills, roles, conflict resolution strategies, reciprocity of need gratification, co-operativeness among network members – should also be assessed.

Network assessment, then, requires that we understand the social needs and capabilities of the older patient, and also who is helping and in what ways.

Recording findings

Having collected a large amount of data through interview, observation, physical examination and network assessment, you must record the data in an accurate, concise and organised way. Recorded data must be readily accessible to other nurses and members of the health care team.[12,22,23]

Employing a standard format for collecting data in the first instance will help to provide some order and reduce the tendency to forget pertinent information. A variety of assessment forms have been developed.[23] The reader is encouraged to contact a Geriatric Assessment Unit to view the particular form in current use. Generally, assessment forms will enable collection of information relating to:

- identifying data
- present health/illness status
- past health
- family health
- personal and social history
- review of systems

The assessment form used by Greenwich Hospital in Sydney, New South Wales, a large geriatric assessment and rehabilitation hospital, appears below.

GREENWICH HOSPITAL NURSING HISTORY

Name____________________ Age__________ Unit No.__________

*Admitting date*____ Time__am/pm *Admitted from:* Home__ Hospital__

Other __________

Diagnosis ____________________ Via: Ambulatory _____

Wheelchair _____

____________________ Stretcher _____

____________________ *Occupation* ____________________

Relevant previous hospitalisation (within past 5-10 years) Place(s) & Date(s)

___

___

Past history: ___

___

___

Reason for admission ___

History obtained from: ___ *History taken by* ___

Date & time taken ___

PHYSICAL

	Yes	No
A. *Mental Status*		
Alert		
Oriented time/place		
Confused		
Apprehensive		
Comatose		
Semi-comatose		
Other		
B. *Physical Traits*		
Deaf: partial/total		
Blind		
Amputee		
Other		
C. *Prosthesis*		
Glasses		
Wigs		
Hearing aid		
Other		
Dentures		
Upper/lower		
Bridge		
Plate		

	Yes	No	Comments
D. *Allergies*			
Drugs			
Food			
Other			
E. *Sleeping Habits*			
Good			
Short naps			
Poor			
Pillows used			
Sedation needed			
F. *Medications*			
Taken prior to admission			
Taken today			
Brought with you			
Sent home			
G. *Safety Precautions*			
Side rails			
Restraints			
Smoking			
Other			

H. *Speech*	Yes	No	Comments
Normal			
Slurred			
Aphasic			
I. *Appetite*			
Good			
Fair			
Poor			
J. *Diet*			
Food restricted			
Feeds self			
Needs assistance			
Alcohol			
Feeding tube			
Likes			
Dislikes			
K. *Mobility*			
Ambulatory			
Needs assistance			
Walking frame			
Crutches			
Cane			
Wheelchair			
Bed			
Other			
L. *Personal Hygiene*			
Shower			
Bath			
Assistance needed			
Cleaning teeth			
M. *Bowels*			
Open daily			
Specify frequency			
Aperients used			
Haemorrhoids			
Incontinent			

Psycho-Social

P. *Communication*	Yes	No
English speaking		
Native language		
Other language		
List		
Q. *Attitude*		
Outgoing		
Responsive		
Fearful		
Withdrawn		
Co-operative		
Other		
R. *Home Environment*		
House		
Unit		
Lift		
Stairs		
Adequate bathroom facilities		

Spiritual

T. Religion

Practising		
Requests		
Chaplain visits		
Prayer/Bible reading		
Religious practices		
Communion		
Last rites		
Other		

	Yes	No	Comments
N. *Bladder* Continent			
Catheter			
Nocturia			
Frequency			
O. *Treatments* Tracheostomy			
Colostomy			
Ileostomy			
self-care			
irrigation			
appliance —type			
Foley catheter			
Dressings			
Other			

Observations Temperature_____ Pulse_____ Resp._____ B.P._____
Urinalysis ______________________________

FRONTAL DORSAL

On the figures circle the location of any reddened areas, rashes, bruises, bed sores, etc. State size, shape.

____

____

____

DRESSINGS:____________________

____

Colour: normal; dusky; cyanotic; jaundiced; pale.
Skin: normal; purpura; bruised; warm; dry; clammy; cold; scars; decubiti; lacerations.
Nail beds: pale; pink; cyanotic.
Lips: pale; pink; cyanotic; cracked; herpes.
Eyes: normal; sunken; discharging; inflamed. *Pupils:* normal; constricted; dilated; fixed.
Mouth: clean; coated; ulcerated; infected; dry.

Specific Symptoms
Pain: Site (specify) ____________________
Characteristics: Mild Moderate Severe Spasmodic Constant
Comments:
____
____
____

Associated with movement? If yes, what? ____________________
Eating ____________________
Breathing/coughing ____________________
Walking ____________________
Other ____________________

Previous management ____________________

Nausea/Vomiting: Frequency: ____________________
Related to food, drugs, activity, other.
Previous management ____________________

Dyspnoea: At rest
On exertion
Mild, moderate, severe
Associated with sputum
Previous management____________________

Sputum: Excessive, minimal.
Colour – white, yellow, green, blood-stained.

Who is the closest confidant? ____________________

Are they available to visit?____________________

With whom does the patient live? ____________________

What has the patient been told about his/her condition or reason for admission? ____________________
____
____

Special requests ____________________
____

Family response to patient's admission ____________________

____

Seen by Doctor
Relative interviewed by Registered Nurse.
Apparent need to contact – Social Worker, Physiotherapist, OT, DT, Chaplain.
Introduced – Self . . Other staff . . Other patients . .
Given information regarding – Call bell . . Radio . . TV . .
Toilet/bathroom . .
Menu/meal times . .
Visiting hours . .
Chaplains . . Phone . .
Valuables . . Smoking . .
Kiosk . . Nightwear . . .
Hairdresser . . Podiatrist . .

Valuables sent home/office ____________________

Summary of Potential Needs or Problems

Physical

____

____

____

____

Psychosocial

____

____

____

Spiritual

____

____

____

(Reproduced with permission)

Nursing diagnosis

Once the nurse has collected all the data about the older person's situation, present and potential nursing care problems must be considered.[5] A statement is then formulated (Nursing Diagnosis) describing these problems and also the patient's strengths and weaknesses. The nursing diagnosis, then, is a statement of a conclusion based on scientific principles and indicates the older person's need for nursing care. It ends the assessment phase and begins the planning phase of the nursing process.[24,25]

There are necessarily similarities between nursing and medical diagnosis. Each begins with the gathering of facts. Then, at some time during or at the conclusion of the fact-gathering, the practitioner recognises a pattern. Both the nursing and medical practitioner then state a conclusion.[5]

Differences in diagnosis arise from each practitioner's view of his role, behaviours and responsibilities and from the knowledge necessary for the practice of each profession. The nurse's view of nursing determines her view of nursing responsibilities and the knowledge these responsibilities require. A nurse can make a nursing diagnosis which specifies an aspect of the patient's condition that requires nursing care. These aspects will exclude health problems for which the accepted mode of therapy is prescription drugs, surgery, radiotherapy and other treatments that are defined legally as the practice of medicine.[26]

Nursing diagnoses in older patient care might include:

- constipation as a result of insufficient bulk in the diet;
- sensory deprivation related to reluctance to wear prescribed glasses;
- dependency on others due to inability to accept wife's recent death;
- sense of powerlessness associated with immobility;
- anxiety related to proposed exploratory surgery.

Obviously, skill in writing nursing diagnoses will come with experience and practice.

Summary

The nursing process can be applied quite readily by the nurse in older patient/client care although some modifications are necessary in the assessment process. A thorough assessment will produce a list of identifiable problems, both actual and potential. From these, nursing diagnoses can be made which will guide the planning and implementation of nursing management.

Questions

1. Why does Bloch depart from the four-step model of the Nursing Process and introduce a fifth step – 'Definition of the problem'?
2. Give five reasons why the assessment process is somewhat different in older adults compared to that in younger adults. What adjustments can the nurse make to accommodate these differences?
3. What are desirable interviewer behaviours?
4. Provide three examples of physical assessment skills under the following headings:
   (a) cardiovascular system
   (b) respiratory system
   (c) abdomen
   (d) eyes
   (e) ears
5. Why is it important to record findings accurately, concisely and in an organised way?
6. What are the advantages of using a standardised assessment format?
7. What is 'Nursing Diagnosis'?

Task

Select a patient or client who is currently experiencing:

- falls, or
- insomnia, or
- constipation, or
- hypothermia, or
- pressure sores, or
- urinary incontinence.

1. Complete a full health and physical status assessment.
2. Identify physical and psychological problems and potential problems.
3. Formulate a nursing diagnosis list of actual and/or potential problems.

4. Select *one* identified problem (see 2 above) and describe the physiological and/or psychosocial bases of the problem.
5. Formulate a nursing objectives list.
6. Outline the rationale for the management of the problem identified (see 4 above).
7. Discuss the use of community resources and the involvement of family members and the patient in his/her care.

Resources: Programmed Instruction Units

1. Mechner F. Patient assessment: examination of the chest and lungs. American Journal of Nursing 1976; 9: 1453-75.
2. Mechner F. Patient assessment: examination of the heart and great vessels: Part 1. American Journal of Nursing 1976; 11: 1807-30.
3. Mechner F. Patient assessment: examination of the eye: Part 1. American Journal of Nursing 1974; 11 suppl. 1-24; Part 2, 1975; 1: 1-24.
4. Mechner F. Patient assessment: examination of the ear. American Journal of Nursing 1975; 3: suppl. 1-24.
5. Mechner F. Patient assessment: auscultation of the heart: Part 2. American Journal of Nursing 1977; 2: 275-98.
6. Mechner F. Patient assessment: examination of the abdomen. American Journal of Nursing 1974; 9: 1679-702.
7. Mechner F. Patient assessment: neurological examination: Part 3. American Journal of Nursing 1976; 4: 609-33.

References

1. Henderson V, Nite G. Principles and practice of nursing. New York: MacMillan Publishing Co. 1978.
2. Hargreaves I. The nursing process. The key to individualised care. Nursing Times 28 Aug. 1975; 89-91.
3. Crow J. The nursing process – 1. Theoretical background. Nursing Times 16 June 1977; 892-896.
4. Humphries MR. The nursing process. An application of scientific method. The Australian Nurses Journal 1979; 9(4): 30-31.
5. Marriner A. The nursing process. St Louis: C.V. Mosby, 1979.
6. Gooch JK. An experience of the nursing process. Nursing Times 5 Feb. 1981; 237-238.

7. McCarthy MM. The nursing process: application of current thinking in clinical problem-solving. Journal of Advanced Nursing, 1981; 6: 173-177.
8. Bloch D. Some crucial terms in nursing: what do they really mean? Nursing Outlook, 1974; 22: 689-694.
9. Eliopoulos C, ed. Health assessment of the older adult. California: Addison-Wesley Publishing Co. 1984.
10. Carotenuto R, Bullock J. Physical assessment of the gerontologic client. Philadelphia: F.A. Davis Co. 1981.
11. Ebersole P, Hess P. Toward healthy aging. St Louis: C.V. Mosby, 1985.
12. Eliopoulos C. Geriatric nursing. London: Harper & Row, 1980.
13. Bates B. A guide to physical assessment. 3rd ed. Philadelphia: J.B. Lippincott Co. 1983.
14. Benjamin A. The helping interview. New York: Prentice-Hall, 1974.
15. de Julia N. The nursing interview. The Australian Nurses Journal, 1980; 10(5); 39.
16. Cameron JE. 'Giant leap forward' begins with the nursing interview. The Australian Nurses Journal, 1982; 12(2): 47-48.
17. Agate J. The practice of geriatrics. London: William Heinemann Medical Books Ltd. 1970.
18. Ham R, Holtzman JM, Marcy ML, Smith MR. Primary care geriatrics. Boston: John Wright, 1983.
19. Brocklehurst JC, Hanley T. Geriatric medicine for students. Edinburgh: Churchill Livingstone, 1981.
20. Cole E. Assessing needs for elders' networks. Journal of Gerontological Nursing, 1985; 11(7): 31-34.
21. Ewing EA. Who cares about Mr D? Journal of Gerontological Nursing, 1984; 10(4): 16-25.
22. Carnevali DL, Patrick M. Nursing management for the elderly. Philadelphia: J.B. Lippincott Co. 1979.
23. McCloskey JC. The nursing care plan. Nursing Forum 1975; 14(4): 364-382.
24. Lunney M. Nursing diagnosis: refining the system. American Journal of Nursing March 1982; 456-459.
25. Wilson G. Nursing diagnosis (assessment) and changing accountability. The Australian Journal of Nursing 1980; 9(10): 36-38.
26. Gordon M. Nursing diagnosis and the diagnostic process. In Chaska NL. The nursing profession: views through the mist. New York: McGraw-Hill, 1978.

Chapter 7

Mental Health and Illness in Old Age

Objectives

To enable the reader to:

1. define and describe the developmental task of old age as identified by Erikson;
2. discuss major theories of psychological ageing;
3. identify and describe organisations and programs which help promote mental and emotional health;
4. explore the crisis of retirement for the elderly;
5. describe factors that influence reactions to retirement;
6. discuss how the older person may be helped to adjust to retirement;
7. identify and evaluate the myths and stereotypes related to sexuality in old age;
8. identify sexual problems in old age and describe their management;
9. describe the causes and manifestations of cognitive and emotional impairment in the elderly;
10. discuss the nursing management of the older person with cognitive and emotional impairment.

Any study of mental health in the older person will include such factors as the psychology and sociology of ageing, mental and emotional health promotion, retirement, sexuality, and mental illness in old age.

Psychology of ageing

Chronological age may not be a reliable index of the older person's mental development, but the initial level of ability would appear to be crucial. It is also crucial for continued learning. Those with a higher IQ are generally able to cope better with current stresses and new situations, and work more effectively in familiar situations by using a variety of skills that are enhanced by experience and maturity. Verbal facility, judgment skills, learning retention and cognitive skills continue into advanced old age because of the brain's tremendous reserve capacity.[1,2]

Generally, the older person is likely to have superior factual knowledge, co-ordination of facts and ideas, life experience and wisdom. Rigidity and concreteness in thought, once considered typical of old age, is rather to be seen as cautiousness.[1,2] There are numerous examples of creative and productive old people.

Psychomotor responses

Older people move more slowly than younger age groups, and precision of response also declines with age. Changes seem to relate to cerebral cortex functioning rather than to any loss of ability to move. Such decline may, to varying degrees, reduce the aged individual's ability to exert control over the environment. Tasks that were formerly not a problem may become so with increasing age. Activities directly related to health maintenance and care may also become more difficult to carry out. These changes have direct implications for community and institutional care of older people.[1,2]

Emotional factors

The older person is generally more apprehensive about new learning situations, especially in a competitive atmosphere, and often cautious because of past experiences. Tasks are often selected, therefore, that have less risk involved or a higher probability of success. The elderly usually have a fairly accurate understanding of their positive and negative characteristics, and are more inclined to like themselves in spite of their faults. If given the opportunity, they will usually try new activities, despite the limitations imposed by impaired physical health and other stressors. They will often cope with stressful and taxing situations better than younger age groups.[1]

Most older people are in contact with their environment and are emotionally mature most of the time.[3] They function adequately in the community, and maintain life roles appropriate to their age without being a nuisance to others.

Behavioural theories of ageing

Historically, psychologists have had little to say about the dynamics of old age. Psychoanalytical theorists focused on developmental theories of childhood and adolescence.[2] Carl Jung was an exception to this in that he was interested in adult personality development. He noted, for example, that introversion became more marked in later life.[3]

Perhaps one of the most important contributions to the understanding of the psychology of ageing has come from Erik Erikson's study of personality development. Erikson's work has helped to modify that of Freud, and other psychoanalytical theorists, by emphasising social factors and placing biological factors in perspective. Erikson identified eight stages of man's personality development and the 'developmental task' inherent in each stage[1,3,4] (see Table 7.1).

Table 7.1 Erikson's Stages of Development

STAGE	1	2	3	4	5	6	7	8
Maturity								Ego integrity vs Despair
Adulthood							Generativity vs Stagnation	
Young Adulthood						Intimacy vs Isolation		
Puberty and Adolescence					Identity vs Role confusion			
Latency				Industry vs Inferiority				
Locomotor-Genital			Initiative vs Guilt					
Muscular-Anal		Autonomy vs Shame, doubt						
Oral Sensory	Basic trust vs Mistrust							

Source: E.H. Erikson, Childhood and Society, New York, Norton, 1964. Reproduced with permission.

Erikson suggested that the development of certain basic attitudes towards others, towards oneself and towards life in general arise in a manner which parallels the development of specialised cells from the undifferentiated mass. During each stage of development, there is a 'developmental task' to be accomplished which contributes some vital outlook or attribute of personality and forms the undergirding for the next stage. If the development of a particular attitude is discouraged, the personality will be deficient in the basic outlook which should have arisen at that critical time.

Erikson identified the developmental task of old age as being the achievement of a sense of ego integrity versus succumbing to a sense of self-despair. The former state involves the person accepting his life as worthwhile. The older person acknowledges that his life *could* have been different although he does not wish it to be different. He recognises that he has made a positive contribution to the world. If this developmental task is not resolved the person feels a sense of despair and self-disgust and is less able to cope with life changes. Life is seen as futile and the aged person may feel there is not enough time left to rectify past mistakes. The older person's feelings of self-disgust and anger may, in turn, be projected onto others.[4,5]

Not all theorists agree with Erikson. Some argue that one must go beyond the recognition of the basic foundation of identity to the possibility of expansion and growth. Others have attempted to refine Erikson's proposals.[3,6]

Sociologists and social psychologists have also addressed the issue of ageing. Role theory, for example, has concentrated on adjustments to the changing roles that accompany the process of ageing. Such adjustments include giving up social relationships and roles typical of adulthood and replacing them with social relationships typical of later years.

Another theory, the 'Activity Theory', emphasises the relationship between activity and life satisfaction in the later years. An early popular theory, known as the 'Disengagement Theory', proposed that the ageing person experiences well-being by disengaging from roles played in society and reducing the number of interactions he has with others. Many studies tested this theory and it was found wanting. Well-being, therefore, seems to go with activity, not disengagement, and one must also take into account the older person's personality structure and state of physical health.[2,4,7]

Personality theorists suggest that there is a relationship between personality and successful ageing. Some research has been undertaken in this area[1,2] but it will not be elaborated on here (see Ebersole and Hess).[3] It has been suggested that there are three, five, or perhaps eight personality types to be found in the aged population. There is some danger in this approach, as personality should not be seen as a fixed system that is completed in childhood. The effect of social environment should not be overlooked as a contributing factor in personality adaptation.

The reader need not accept any of the theories presented here in totality. Each adds its own contribution to our better understanding of the older person.

Ageing – a dynamic process

Ageing may be seen as a dynamic process in which the older person never reaches a point where he can say 'This is me' or 'I have arrived'. The older person, therefore, may be seen as in a continual state of becoming.[3,8] He continues to learn about himself in the world, is aware of his own and others' emotional needs, wants to direct his own destiny, and tries to find a meaningful and comfortable fit between the self and society. There are some old people who will become more of what they were. If they were hard to live with when younger, they may be harder to live with in old age. Personality characteristics in the older person may thus be seen as an exaggeration of lifelong personality traits.

Personality development will have been affected throughout the older person's life by many variables. These include health status, sociocultural background, group membership, social identity, role opportunity, birth order, family dynamics, ability to satisfy needs, general living situation and motivation.[1-3,5] To complicate this picture, it is suggested that an interaction of variables occurs. The more favourably older people 'score' on these variables, the more likely they will be to have a wider range of behaviours and to be more adaptive. Although some become cantankerous, others mellow and become more tolerant. The latter have probably achieved adequate gratification during their life and successfully mastered disappointments. The former are likely to have many unmet needs and a low frustration tolerance.[8] Even so, the view is taken here that they are still capable of personal growth, although some will need help to realise their potential.

Older people have much to draw upon – past experiences, memories and relationships.[3] If these have been positive and personally rewarding, then this is likely to prove helpful in old age. Unfortunately, many older people do not have these advantages and, the longer they live, the more they may lose the beneficial effect of what they did have. Also, older people have to cope with multiple stresses while experiencing major changes socially, physically and psychologically.[3] Lowered expectations of older persons, by others, may also influence their will to cope.

Throughout life, adjustments are made as the individual ages chronologically. The realisation that one is ageing usually occurs in middle age or earlier, as evidence of bodily and social changes becomes more apparent. Some find these changes devastating, while others readily adapt. Typical factors which prompt adjustment include approaching retirement, reduced income, decreased levels of health, changes in relationships, and the inevitability of approaching death.[3] The older person, then, is faced with a wide variety of stressors. Response will be influenced by a number of factors, including personality and the degree of threat perceived.[3]

Mental and emotional health in old age

Mental and emotional health in old age may be promoted in a variety of ways. There follows a description of some of the organisations and programs which may help to reduce the stresses of old age. The list is not exhaustive. It may be difficult for some old people to take up the opportunities available. Others will need to be made aware of their existence and encouraged and helped to participate, although this will not always be easy.

1. **School for Seniors.** This organisation was established in 1969 in the Wesley Centre, Pitt Street, Sydney. It has the motto 'While I live We'll learn'. Classes are held twice weekly and include academic subjects, hobby type classes, and special demand classes (e.g. lip reading, dancing, choir). Fees are nominal and gain entry to as many classes as desired. The Volunteer Social Committee promotes theatre visits, bus outings, live-in conferences, and holidays.

2. **Senior Australians for Growth and Exploration** (SAGE) originated in the United States in 1974 and began in Sydney in 1980. It evolved to help people of retirement age to experience new dimensions of growth, spontaneity and learning. In three-hourly sessions, at weekly intervals, over a period of twelve weeks, facilitators and members take part in 'socially enjoyable, non-threatening exercises which include relaxation, deep breathing, communication, stress management and creative sharing'. Close relationships within the group are aimed at and this helps to break down barriers of isolation and loneliness.

3. **SPAN** is a co-operative of older and retired people, sharing their skills in the community. It was initiated by the Brotherhood of St Laurence, a non-government welfare agency, in Melbourne, Australia, with the intention of demonstrating what could be done to change the community's attitude towards the aged. The programs of SPAN are an example of older people as the service providers, rather than the recipients. Through the programs, older people are able to 'pass on the skills acquired during their lifetime, to learn new ones, and to widen their relationship opportunities'. These activities are grouped under craft, reading, home handyman service, community education and social action.[9]

4. **Evening Colleges.** These are conducted by the Department of Education, usually during the evening. Courses are available in crafts, languages and leisure interests.[10]

5. **New South Wales Department of Technical and Further Education** (TAFE). The department has many colleges throughout New South Wales and a College of External Studies which offers some correspondence courses.[10]

6. **Workers Educational Association** (WEA). This offers a wide range of courses for older people.[10]

7. **Beehive Industries.** This is a centre in Sydney where older people who have left the workforce spend a few hours each day working in a no-pressure atmosphere. There are also recreation and leisure activities available.

8. **Healthcraft.** Many community health centres are running Healthcraft programs. These aim to increase older people's knowledge about health issues, and suggest ways of improving their health and enhancing their life. Programs address a number of questions which are of interest to the elderly, such as: what happens as we age; how the health system works; relaxation; coping with stress; how to appreciate getting older; and new ideas for leisure activities.

9. **Healthy Lifestyle Vacations.** These vacations were introduced by the New South Wales Health Department in 1982 and have since been adopted by other states. The project is a 5-day residential holiday with health promotion activities encompassing the physical, mental and social aspects of health and fitness.

10. **Foster Grandparent Scheme.** Foster grandparents have been employed by state government residential institutions for mentally retarded children. Each person 'adopts' one or more children and, working within the institution, gives them something of the continued love and support that would normally come from a grandparent in normal family life.[11]

11. **Senior Citizens Clubs.** There are many groups and clubs for the elderly in Australia. Senior Citizens Clubs are only one example. These clubs offer varied social activities, including card playing, old-time dancing, carpet bowls, socialising, entertainment, coach tours, concerts and holidays. There is often a free lending library at these centres.

Retirement

In Australia, it is common practice for men to retire at sixty-five and women at sixty. These are the prescribed retiring ages in many jobs and are the ages for old age pension eligibility.[12] There are, however, indications that increasing numbers of men retire at sixty or less and women at fifty-five. These men and women will obviously spend a longer period of time outside the workforce.

Retirement is a major turning point in adult development. It is a crisis which can threaten a person's feelings of identity, integrity and self-esteem. For most it will mean 'loss or reduction of income, influences, authority, status, social relationships, professional skills, creativity, activity, and control over the environment'.[8] These changes, combined with the physical changes associated with the ageing process, may affect the older person's personality and his sense of self-worth. Emotions, health and sexual relationships may also be affected.[3,13,14]

Retirement is probably more of a crisis for the man, although there is no doubt that women are affected too, and will become increasingly so as their participation in the workforce increases. Most women, however, have had to remain flexible because of the constant role modifications and crises associated with bearing and rearing children, homemaking and career that they have had to undergo throughout their adult life.

People retire for varying reasons. Early retirement may be voluntary or involuntary. Others retire at the prescribed age unwillingly. Illness may be a contributing factor in early retirement, and those who retire at sixty or sixty-five years of age may also have serious health problems. Many will have adequate finances on retirement, others will not. Feelings of relative deprivation associated with illness, financial insecurity or compulsory retirement may generate other problems for the older person which will need to be resolved to ensure a satisfactory retirement. Usually, preparation for retirement has been absent or inadequate.[3]

The individual who has been obsessively tied to work will obviously experience a strong sense of loss on retirement. The perfectionist with rigid standards, who has difficulty accepting himself and his accomplishments, may also experience difficulties.[3] Many others will not have developed hobbies, interests or friendships over the years before retirement.

Income is one of the basic concerns of the older person who is facing retirement or has already retired.[15] The value of savings is eroded by inflation as the cost of living continues to rise. Some retired people feel guilty about receiving 'welfare payments' from the government, and society is ambivalent in its attitude towards the older person receiving a pension. Lack of information and planning prevents many from enjoying all the benefits available.[16] Others experience inadequate income which affects the availability of housing, health care, transportation, activities, food and home maintenance. Conversely, wisely invested savings and adequate pensions contribute to a positive adjustment to retirement.[17]

We can now identify some of the factors that affect a satisfactory retirement. These include:

- adequate finances;
- reasonable health;

- pressures to retire;
- attitudes towards retirement;
- personality characteristics.

To this list, Ebersole and Hess[3] add:

- employability;
- level of information about retirement.

Nursing roles relating to retirement

The nurse will find herself relating to the older person who is about to retire or has retired in the context of the person's home, or in the hospital, or in factories and businesses. Nurses, however, have rarely addressed the issue of nursing function related to retirement.

Nurses should be aware that major changes in a person's life, such as retirement, are likely to be reflected in their physical, psychological and social status.[3] The nurse may be able to identify problem areas and instil hope by encouraging insight into the transitory stress caused by retirement. Stressors that add to the chaotic feelings associated with retirement should be identified.[1,3,16] The nurse can help the person involved to examine how he has coped with crises in the past. The strengths identified can be reinforced and weaknesses supported. The retired person can be encouraged to review his work experience and its meaning for him.[3]

Nurse counselling in relation to retirement might focus on income, activities, living arrangements, role change, and legal issues.[3] Obviously, some of these matters will be beyond the scope of the nurse and a knowledge of the availability of pre-retirement planning programs will be helpful.[18,19] These are available through a number of agencies, such as:

- banks;
- insurance companies;
- Public Service Board;
- Council on the Ageing;
- superannuation boards.

Planning in financial, social and emotional areas will promote better adjustment.[20] Realisation of the potential and rewards of retirement can aid that adjustment. The retired person is freed from the constraints of routine and employment and there is now sufficient time to do those things that a life of regular work precluded. Retirees are free to enter voluntary work, leisure, recreational and cultural activities. The nurse must remember, though, that freedom can sometimes be quite threatening to the patient or client she is managing. Acceptance of government financial benefits should be encouraged and any negative or ambivalent feelings associated with this freely discussed.

As part of retirement intervention, older individuals should be encouraged to establish and practise good health habits.[10] Proper diet, avoidance of alcohol, drugs and tobacco, and regular physical exercise and examinations are to be encouraged.[10,21] For those who wish to move house after retirement, the nurse can help her client to explore such things as the cost of living and the availability of services and health care, before making such a move.[3] The effect of retirement on the retiree's spouse may be unexpectedly negative because of the sudden increase of interpersonal exposure. Wives, for example, may find their social arrangements interrupted because of pressures, subtle or otherwise, to fit in with their husband's plans. If she is still working, she may feel coerced into retiring earlier than planned or desired.[3,22] The nurse can indicate to couples the need to spend time apart from each other.

Sexuality

Not too long ago, human sexuality was seen as an activity that was important only to the young. Society, to a large extent, felt that the ageing adult was asexual, unable, or uninterested in sexuality.[23] The older person may unthinkingly have adopted these views and developed a negative self-image as a sexual being.[24] Over the past few years, however, research has dispelled the myths about sexual activity in later life.[25] In the mid 1960s, Masters and Johnson popularised the startling notion that ageing people can and do enjoy sexual expression.[26]

Generally, research indicates that there is no physiological reason for the cessation of sexual relations in older persons.[23-25] Sexuality is an important component of life at all ages. We must remember, though, that sexuality involves a wide variety of behaviour, not just the act of sexual intercourse itself. Holding hands, touching in other ways, kissing and masturbation are only some of the many ways in which sexuality may be expressed.[3,25]

It is, perhaps, the older person who is most in need of sexual comfort because of the losses that characterise the ageing experience in our society. The ability to give and receive sexually is really a re-affirmation of oneself as an attractive, worthwhile and important human being.

Sexual problems

Increasing age brings with it a number of changes, many of which have an impact on sexuality. Various writers,[1,3,23-27] have identified a number of anatomical and physiological changes in old age:

For women

- altered body contour;
- change in reproductive capability;
- cessation of menses;
- decrease in vaginal length and width;
- decreased vaginal lubrication related to thinning and drying of the vaginal mucosa;
- reduction in Bartholin gland secretion;
- inability of the vagina to secrete acid, leading to a greater tendency for vaginal infections;
- loss of elasticity in the vaginal walls;
- vaginal burning, pelvic aching, pain during intercourse related to changes noted.

For men

- fertility does not cease with age;
- the older male requires more time and direct genital stimulation to achieve an erection;
- the intensity of the ejaculatory experience diminishes;
- an erection is harder to maintain;
- the time interval between ejaculations tends to increase.

Sexual problems may also be related to diseases such as coronary artery disease, diabetes mellitus, alcoholism, hypo- and hyperthyroidism and arthritis. Drugs (e.g. antihypertensives, tranquillisers, steroids, antidepressants), surgery (e.g. prostatectomy), senile vaginitis, malnutrition, anaemia, and respiratory, genitourinary, neurological and infectious disorders may also cause problems.[3,23-25,27-30]

Other factors influencing sexual expression in the older person may be described as psychological in origin. These include feelings of guilt and shame at maintaining sexuality into old age. Misconceptions, such as beliefs that sexual activity is not possible after a hysterectomy, prostatectomy, or cardiac disorder, may also inhibit sexual enjoyment. A more practical problem may be the lack of a partner. For others, it is the lack of privacy, especially where the older person is living with their family, or in a nursing home or hospital.

Perhaps the greatest sexual problem for males is erectile dysfunction. Although organicity may be a contributing factor, psychological factors are most commonly responsible for this problem. Loss of interest and erectile dysfunction may be related to boredom, fatigue, overeating, excessive drinking, psychiatric disabilities (e.g. major depressive disorder)[3,23,31] and the attitudes of society and family. The older person's self-esteem may be affected by the many losses experienced; for example, loss of job and possibly income, declining physical strength and attractiveness, or loss of spouse or long-term friend.

For the older female, loss of a spouse or suitable partner is a major difficulty in continuing to be sexually active. The older female is particularly disadvantaged as she tends to live longer than the male. She is also handicapped more by social mores, and is less able to take the initiative in dating or sexual matters. Finally, she is less likely to marry a younger man.[23,24,29]

All these changes may lead to problems in the sexual relationship, and open and frank communication between partners should be one of the first steps advocated. Specific approaches could include:

- assessment and management of physical disabilities;[25,29]
- assessment of sexual knowledge;[23-25]
- use of artificial lubricants;[3,23,32]
- prolonging the sexual act to provide greater opportunity for each partner to attain sexual gratification;[3]
- increasing use of masturbation;[3,23,25,26]
- oral-genital techniques;
- acceptance of modified forms of sexual behaviour (e.g. caressing, kissing, other physical contact);
- learning to accept changes.[3,23,25,29]

Nursing roles related to sexuality in old age

The nurse has a responsibility to help maintain the sexuality of the older person, and part of the nursing history will include the sexual history.[23] This should be done privately and tactfully, and confidentiality should be fully maintained. The physical examination should have included the reproductive system.[3]

Aged couples can be helped to understand the cultural pressures placed on them.[24,25] The nurse can disseminate information to other professionals, the general public, and the aged themselves. To help the older person, the nurse must be aware of the various physical and psychological causes of sexual dysfunctioning. She must be aware of the various modes of treatment, and must be willing to see sexuality as an important component of the older age group.[1,23,25,26]

The older person experiencing erectile dysfunction will need reassurance that this does not necessarily mean that sexual function is lost forever.

The possible causes of such dysfunction should be explained to both partners, and the patient should be examined by his doctor. If there is an organic problem which cannot be corrected, the possible implantation of a penile prosthesis may be explored.[1,3,31]

Whenever possible, health problems should be identified and corrected. Specific information about the capacities and limitations of sexual activity in the light of any existing health problem is an important aspect of patient education. Counselling regarding the effects of poor diet and alcohol on sexual activity should be undertaken where applicable. Such basic education can help the aged to understand the effects of the ageing process on sexuality by providing a realistic framework for sexual functioning.[3,23,25]

Consideration must be given to the sexual needs of older people in nursing homes and other institutions. The aged in these situations have a right to privacy. In practical terms they should be able to close and lock a door, feeling secure that this action will be respected. It is obviously a basic courtesy to knock on a person's door before entering their room. Staff should not make clients feel guilty or foolish because of their expressions of love and sexuality.

Masturbation is beneficial in releasing sexual tensions and maintaining continued sexual function and is, generally speaking, not to be discouraged. The nurse can convey acceptance and understanding of the value of this activity. This will help allay feelings of guilt and depression. Staff members in institutions may need to deal with their own anxieties about patients' use of this activity.[3,23,24,26]

Where physical health conditions interfere directly or indirectly with sexual activity, nurses can suggest position changes to alleviate some of the problems.[23,32] Hip surgery to alleviate joint immobility associated with arthritis may help. For those troubled by pain, taking medication before the anticipated sexual activity may help. For problems of fatigue, sexual activity in the morning or after a rest may be helpful.[3,32]

Cardiovascular disease can also interfere with sexual expression. Generally, sexual activity is resumed slowly after a myocardial infarction. How soon after should be discussed with the patient's doctor. As strength returns, increased sexual activity is possible. Instruction about position changes may be necessary. The person with coronary disease should be informed of the danger signs (angina, shortness of breath, tiredness, irregular heart beat and tightness in the chest).[30] A Holter Monitor may be useful at times to check for arrhythmias during intercourse. The partner of the person who has had a stroke may fear causing another. Simple instruction on how to decrease anxiety and strain during sexual activity will help to alleviate these fears. It may be necessary for the male stroke patient to change from a top to bottom position. One of the unwanted side effects of the antihypertensive drugs prescribed after a stroke is erectile dysfunction. This should be reported to the patient's doctor so that medication can be reviewed.[3,23,25,32]

Nurses and sex counsellors should examine their own social biases about aged sexuality and increase their understanding of elderly sexual function in order to foster a supportive climate for healthy sexual activity in elderly clients. Full and frank discussion in team meetings might help this to occur, as would inservice education courses.[3,24,26]

Mental illness in old age

Mental illness can occur at any age, but there are some illnesses which are more common in particular age groups, and there are illnesses which by definition occur only in a particular age group.[33,34]

Emotional disorders in the older person may range from mild anxiety to some form of dementia and include the whole range of psychiatric disorders. As well as causing misery to the victim, these illnesses also bring worry and anxiety to relatives, friends, neighbours, family doctors and other professionals.

Emotional disorders of older people may be divided into two groups. Firstly, those illnesses which begin before the age of sixty-five and continue to be a problem into old age and, secondly, those illnesses which begin after the age of sixty-five.[35]

The first group includes:

- the schizophrenic whose illness has gone on unremittingly into old age;
- the schizophrenic who has recovered from attacks in earlier years and then has a relapse in old age;
- the manic depressive who has had previous episodes of illness;
- the alcoholic and drug addict of young or middle-age onset;
- the person with recurrent neurotic illness;[35]
- the individual with a personality disorder which does not become a significant problem until old age (e.g. the person who manages to live an isolated 'schizoid' lifestyle until old age, when disability forces him to live in a group setting);[36]
- the pre-senile dementias;
- dementia due to cerebrovascular disease;
- head injuries and other conditions affecting the brain tissue itself, with or without disease of other organs of the body.[35]

Mental illnesses developing after sixty-five years of age include:

- senile dementia (of the Alzheimer's type);
- the affective psychoses;

- organic brain syndrome due to cerebrovascular disease (multi-infarct dementia);
- schizophrenia (paranoid type, mostly paraphrenia).

Transient situational disturbances are quite common after sixty-five, although psychoneurotic illness developing in this age group is rare. Where late onset alcoholism and drug dependence occurs, it is usually secondary to another illness. Acute brain syndrome (delirium) is another problem experienced by this age group and when it does occur the person is most frequently admitted to a general hospital for treatment.[33-36]

Several of the more common disorders occurring in old age are described below.

Dementia

Dementia is a clinical term for a varied group of neurological diseases affecting intellect, memory, emotions, behaviour, personality and social functioning. It exists where there is sufficient damage (or impairment) of enough of the brain so that the person can no longer function effectively. (The cut-off point, however, is always a problem.) These diseases have differing aetiologies and clinical features which are often specific for the individual disease processes.

Senile dementia of the Alzheimer's type, and multi-infarct dementia, comprise over 90 per cent of all dementias.[3,33,34,36] Established dementia is present in 5 per cent of the community aged sixty-five years and over and in 20 per cent aged eighty years and over.[37] Many would say that there should be no routine tests for dementia in certain older patients (e.g. an 88-year-old lady with five years of established dementia). However, dementia may be reversible (see DSM III for a discussion of this concept). It is important, therefore, to make an accurate early diagnosis. Routine screening could include a range of tests:

- blood tests to determine the levels of:
  - serum electrolytes and urea
  - liver function
  - calcium and phosphate
  - vitamin B_{12} and folate
  - haemoglobin
  - ESR
- serology for syphilis
- thyroid function
- chest X-ray

- EEG
- micro-urine test
- random blood sugar
- CAT scan
- ECG
- lumbar puncture (occasionally).[3,33,34,36]

Non-reversible dementia

Non-reversible dementias in the older person include:

- senile dementia of the Alzheimer's type (SDAT);
- multi-infarct dementia (MID);
- the dementias associated with Parkinson's disease and multiple sclerosis;
- Huntington's disease.[33,34,36]

Senile dementia of the Alzheimer's type

The majority of the elderly have senile dementia of the Alzheimer's type (SDAT). It is characterised by generalised shrinkage of the cerebral cortex. It occurs in twice as many women as men. Genetic and social, environmental and personality factors are involved in the development of the illness.[33,34,36] Hypotheses include:

- selective cell death caused by viral or environmental agents;[33,38]
- excessive accumulation of aluminium or other toxins;[38]
- a genetic defect;[33,36,38]
- an age-related change in the immune system;[38]
- reduction in the acetylcholine-mediated transmission of nerve impulses.[39]

The clinical picture of SDAT is characterised by:[33,34,36,40]

- insidious onset
- steady progression
- early and progressive amnesia
- aphasia
- apraxia
- agnosia

- motor system disorder
- loss of insight } minor features
- apathy/inertia }

Late onset SDAT (75 years plus) may have a different clinical pattern, with less striking apraxia and agnosia, and more cognitive slowing, apathy and inertia.[40]

As yet, no drug exists that can cure SDAT, although some very promising work is being carried out with substances which increase acetylcholine activity.[41] Tranquillisers may relieve concurrent agitation or hostility and antidepressants will help relieve reactive depression.[34,36] Other management will involve social and milieu therapy and a balance between structured routines and fresh activities. Ideally, the person suffering from SDAT should be maintained in the community for as long as possible, as removal often leads to confusion and further disturbed behaviour.[33,34,36,42]

Multi-infarct dementia

Here dementia is related to arterial disease of the brain. There are two major types of MID:

- large vessel disease – with emboli from platelet thrombi and atheromatous plaques. Where dementia results from several large infarcts the diagnosis is usually clear from the start and their presence will be seen on a CAT scan. Treatment with anticoagulants (including Aspirin) will sometimes be attempted;[33,34,36,40]
- small vessel disease – disease of the small vessels (arterioles) with a tendency to get small infarcts and to produce a 'lacunar state' (emotional lability, dysarthria, ataxia, marche à petits pas [walk with little steps]). Treatment of underlying conditions (e.g. hypertension, diabetes mellitus) is important.[33,34,36,40]

Caring for the carer

Looking after someone with dementia becomes difficult and exhausting for the carer as time goes by. Problems facing the carer will include time demands, isolation from others, and management of their own and the sufferer's affairs. Day-night reversal, belligerence by the sufferer, wandering behaviour, change of role, and 'dangerous behaviour' may also create problems.[43,44]

Support in such a situation has to be realistic and include practical advice. Williams *et al*[45] suggest the following issues will require attention:

- home care
- domiciliary care benefits
- respite care
- financial and legal advice
- sitting services
- nursing home accommodation
- architectural and security advice
- coping with the dementing person

Alzheimer's Disease and Related Disorders Society (ADARDS) is a self-help organisation for relatives, friends and sufferers from dementia. It provides support by holding regional meetings, arranging outings and mutual minding groups, and establishing networks and domiciliary services.

Existing services for the carer and the demented person include:

- Home care – here someone comes in to help with the housework and leaves the carer free to attend to the affected person or take time off;
- Day care centres – sufferers can be left at a centre where they will be supervised, cared for and involved in stimulating activities by professional staff;
- Holiday care (respite care) – the sufferer is looked after in a hospital or nursing home so as to allow the regular carer a much needed break or holiday.[38]

Reversible dementia

Dementia may be progressive, static or remitting.[46] Many older people who present with clinical signs of dementia do not, in fact, have irreversible pathology of the central nervous system. The loss of functional capacity may be secondary to some treatable pathophysiological or emotional state.[34] Causes may include:

- drug effects
- trauma
- infection
- anaemias
- metabolic disorder
- neoplastic disease
- depression
- isolation
- translocation shock
- thyroid disorders

- diseases of the heart and lungs
- renal and hepatic insufficiency
- vitamin B_{12} and folate deficiency
- normal pressure hydrocephalus
- visual and hearing disorders
- pain
- alcohol[3,33,34,36,47–49]

The phenomenon of reversible dementia underscores the need for complete physical, psychological and laboratory investigations of patients with cognitive dysfunction.

Delirium

Delirium is more common in the elderly than any other age group. It always has an underlying cause, most commonly some insult to the body (see above for examples). Other causes may be emotional in origin.

Delirium may be characterised by a fluctuating clouding of consciousness, disorientation, agitation, hallucinosis and fear. Clouding of consciousness readily allows for misinterpretation of ordinary events. Delirium is often worse at night, when delusions are common, particularly those of persecution. The hallucinations are visual and frightening. Some degree of restlessness is also usual. On the other hand, delirium can be a quiet phenomenon, without agitation, hallucinosis or fear.[3,33,34,36]

Failure to make an accurate assessment may result in the older person being treated as someone suffering from dementia, with all the consequences of this diagnosis. Every effort should be made to prevent the development of delirium and to treat it rapidly and effectively if it has occurred already. The response to treatment will depend on the cause, the magnitude of the effect on the sufferer, and the overall state of health of the patient.[33,34,36]

Nursing care in dementia

Activities of daily living

The older person who is clean, well-groomed and appropriately dressed is more likely to maintain self-esteem. Dyspraxia may interfere with bathing throughout the illness and necessitate supervision by relatives or the nurse. In the latter stages of the illness, it may not be wise to leave the patient alone in the bathroom or toilet and, in particular, the temperature of the bath or shower should be closely monitored. Non-slip bath mats and bath seats will help to prevent accidents. Handrails in the bathroom and toilet will assist the activities of daily living in these areas.

Clothing should be easy, appropriate, comfortable and, if possible, familiar. Special provision may be necessary for the incontinent patient.[3,43,44,50]

Mealtimes and nutrition

Meals should be simple and well-balanced. Nursing care will involve close observation of mealtimes and encouragement to eat. On occasions, the diet will need to be supplemented to provide sufficient nutrition. Drinking will need to be encouraged to prevent dehydration which would otherwise cause more confusion. As eating becomes more difficult due to dyspraxia, various protective devices and practical aids will become increasingly useful.[3,43,44,50]

Constipation and incontinence

Prolonged constipation should give rise to concern. Not only does it cause discomfort but it might also result in more confusion, irritability and perhaps aggressive behaviour. Faecal incontinence may mislead the nurse to miss the fact that the older patient is impacted with faeces. Intervention will include:

- introducing food with high fibre;
- activating the patient;
- adequate fluid intake.

More radical interventions should only be used as a last resort.

There are numerous causes of incontinence in the older age group, so it is important to identify correctly the specific cause in each patient (see Chapter 8 for a discussion of these). It is not good enough simply to accept incontinence as part of the dementing picture. Intervention will involve:

- regular toileting;
- ensuring the older person knows where the toilets are;
- providing ready access to a commode or urine bottle at night;
- responding quickly to the older person's call to go to the toilet.

Where the incontinence is intransigent, protective devices will be helpful. A range of products are available including pads and diapers, protective underpants, disposable drawsheets and washable seat covers for chairs.[3,43,44,50]

Safety

Appliances and furniture should be made as safe as possible. Safety hazards in the garden must also be considered. Anticipation and observation are important nursing interventions here. Night wandering might be a particular problem. Interventions might include:

- closing bedroom doors;
- night-light provision to reduce misperception of stimuli and prevent accidents occurring;
- a bell on exit doors;
- relocation of locks.[3,43,44,50]

Leisure activities

Exercise will improve circulation, respiration and sleep. Other activities should be familiar, easily understood and within the demented person's capabilities. These could include gardening, short car and bus trips, and music. It is important that activities are planned, regular and unhurried.[3,43,44,50]

Medical care

It is important for the nurse to be aware of any change in the demented older person's behaviour. Changes may be due to some illness which needs attention. Importantly, the change may be related to the medication the patient is on. Physical illness and medications may, in fact, exacerbate the clinical features of dementia. Changes should therefore be identified promptly and reported quickly to the patient's doctor.[50]

Memory loss

Although the older person's illness is progressive and permanent, many practical steps can be taken to help them function a little better. Memory may be assisted by:

- repetition of information;
- giving information in a simple format;
- regularity of routine;
- providing large clocks and calendars in clear view;
- providing pictorial representations of bedroom, toilet and bathroom on appropriate doors;
- listing daily activities on a central notice board;
- encouraging photographs of family members.[3,43,44,50]

Problems in communication

As language skills deteriorate in dementia, the nurse will need to become more sensitive to other cues. Over time, she can learn to interpret accurately the older patient's needs when expressed in more non-verbal ways. The nurse's communication in this context should be characterised by simple words and sentences which are spoken slowly and deliberately. These may need to be repeated and it is important that the nurse waits for a response.[3,50]

Disorders of thinking and perception

The experience of delusions and hallucinations may be frightening indeed. Arguing about their absence of any basis in reality will be fruitless and may only compound the problem. Nor should the nurse agree with them as this will only reinforce adherence to them. Rather, the nurse should recognise them for what they are and seek to divert the patient's attention onto something more profitable.[51-53]

Emotional problems

Sudden mood changes are common in dementia and there does not seem to be any identifiable cause. When the demented older patient is over-taxed by demands or situations beyond his ability to cope with, he may respond with anger, aggression, abuse or resistance. This is called a catastrophic reaction. Touch (arm around the shoulder, hand on shoulder, holding or shaking hands) may produce a more positive response. The nurse may also seek to change the subject, distract the older person, or remove him from the stressful situation. It is important for the nurse to remain calm and seek to reassure the patient during the disturbing episode. Obviously, this will not be easy.

Older people may react to their illness with various levels of depression, and severe depression may cause serious physical problems for the elderly. It is important to recognise promptly, therefore, that the person is depressed so that treatment can be implemented as quickly as possible.[33,34,36,50] The confused older person with severe memory loss may experience anxiety about responsibilities in the past (things at home, at work, in the community). It is important to assure them that their feelings are understood and, again, distraction is a useful technique to employ.

Depression in the elderly

Unquestionably, the most common treatable cause of reversible dementia is depression. The term 'depression' encompasses a variety of emotional reactions that range from grief to severe depression.[33-35]

Neurotic and reactive depressions are prevalent among the elderly. The more severe depressions present a clinical picture that is often mistaken for dementia ('pseudo-dementia').[33,34,36] The patient is characteristically withdrawn, neglects himself, expresses odd delusional beliefs, becomes restless at night and during the day, and thinking and actions are slowed. Important clues to the correct diagnosis include the length of the illness, the sad expression and psychomotor retardation.[54]

In this illness, women are more commonly affected than men. The elderly male, it must be noted, has the highest successful suicide rate of both sexes of any age, regardless of the diagnosis.[55,56] Onset may be gradual or sudden. The person has a depressed mood which may improve as the day progresses. Other features include early morning wakening, anorexia, weight loss, preoccupation with bodily symptoms and anxiety. Suicidal thoughts may be based on feelings of sin, guilt, poverty, unworthiness and wrongdoing. Thoughts and actions may be considerably slowed down.[3,33,34,36]

Manic depressive psychosis mostly has its onset before the age of sixty-five but it is not uncommon for it to occur in old age.[55] Age is no barrier to treatment of depression and most older people respond well to antidepressants, anti-manic medication and/or electroconvulsive therapy. Medications include:

- tricyclic antidepressants
- monoamine oxidase inhibitors
- tetracyclic antidepressants
- lithium carbonate

In general, tricyclic antidepressants (e.g. Amitriptyline, Doxepin) are the preferred treatment for depressive illness.[55] Lithium is useful in manic-depressive psychosis, but toxicity can be a problem, especially with unreliable taking of the drug, as can dehydration, fever or interaction with other medication (e.g. diuretics). Monoamine oxidase inhibitors (e.g. Phenelzine, Tranylcypromine) are effective in some patients although their use carries greater risk from interactions with certain foods.[33,34,36,56] Anxiolytics are useful for mild depression and anxiety states.

Nursing care

Nursing care of depressed people will centre around a number of issues.

Provision of a safe environment

This task will be challenging and at times difficult to achieve but it is of the utmost importance to the older person's safety. Sharp instruments, belts and ties, panes of glass may be used by the elderly to inflict serious injury upon themselves. Medications may be secretly hoarded. The nurse will need to be observant and anticipate problems before they occur. This should be done in such a way as to indicate the nurse's concern for the older person's welfare and not as a form of punishment.[52,53]

Provision of personal hygiene

Although depressed people may appear able to do things for themselves, more often than not they are incapable of doing very much. They should not, therefore, be forced or nagged to take part in activities. The nurse may, in fact, have to do most things for the older person who is depressed or at least supervise them closely if they are still able to do some things for themselves.

These activities may include care of body cleanliness, mouth care, grooming and dressing. The closeness of nursing care associated with these activities may contribute significantly to the recovery of patients. As recovery begins, they should be increasingly included in activities.[51,53]

Encouraging sleep

The importance of sleep to recovery cannot be underestimated. The presence of the nurse may help the depressed older person to go to sleep more easily. Talking to the older person, the therapeutic use of touch (see Chapter 4), and teaching relaxation techniques may also be helpful approaches.[3,53]

Monitoring intake and output

The older patient who does not eat or drink because of severe depression poses particular nursing care problems. Encouraging the patient to eat smaller meals and to drink small quantities of fluids may all help to prevent subnutrition, dehydration and constipation.[52,53]

Building meaningful communication patterns

It is important for the nurse to understand accurately the verbal and non-verbal communication behaviours of the older depressed patient. This establishes a baseline from which the nurse can begin to build meaningful communication patterns with the patient.[53] The nurse is strategically placed to teach depressed patients new communication responses which will enable them to express their thoughts and feelings more therapeutically.

Activities to meet psychological needs

Involvement in various activities around the ward can be therapeutic. It may help to expend energy, focus attention on the patient's contribution, and provide meaning for the patient. Occupational therapy will also be helpful in these ways. Encouragement and active recognition are important nursing activities.[51,53]

Mania

Mania occurs less frequently than depression and may occur either before or after a depressive illness, or quite independently of it. The major tranquillisers are used in this situation with good effect.[33,35,36]

Paranoid psychosis (paraphrenia)

Although uncommon, paranoid psychosis is a major problem where it occurs. Pitt[33] describes the older person with paranoid psychosis as being typically 'female, solitary, partially deaf and eccentric, but without a past history of serious psychiatric illness'. It occurs in perhaps one per cent of the population over sixty-five years of age.

Here the older person starts to build up great suspicions about others. Later, auditory hallucinations and persecutory or grandiose delusions occur. The intellect, personality and memory are usually unimpaired.[33,34] Diagnosis of paranoid illness may be open to abuse, so allegations and circumstances need to be critically examined.[33]

Untreated, the illness runs a chronic, unremitting course. Relocation of accommodation sometimes helps for a while. Hospitalisation may become a necessity.[36] Argument with the older person so afflicted is mostly fruitless. Unfortunately, because of the nature of the illness, compliance with medication is particularly difficult. Where it is accepted, phenothiazine tranquillisers produce excellent results and prognosis is related to their maintenance.[33]

Summary

In the past, inaccurate assumptions and beliefs about changes in old age have been held by society at large. The last twenty years or so have been more enlightened but there are still many areas of adult development that have been only minimally explored. The numerous assaults on old age are now recognised. Retirement is a potential crisis period because it is a major turning point in adult development. These assaults, combined with physical changes, may affect various areas of the older person's life, including sexual relations and mental well-being generally. Various organisations and opportunities exist to help keep the older person mentally healthy.

The nurse, whether in the hospital, nursing home or community, has a number of identifiable roles to play in relation to retirement, sexuality, the promotion of mental health and caring for older people with major psychosocial problems.

Questions

1. 'Well-being for the older person comes as she/he reduces the number of interactions and roles in society.' Discuss this statement.
2. What contribution did Erikson make to our understanding of the older person?
3. Name six variables which affect personality development throughout life.
4. Describe three opportunities for mental health promotion.
5. List six stressors that a person has to face in old age.
6. Describe six effects of retirement.
7. What 'individual' factors affect the older person's response to retirement?
8. How may the nurse help the older person to prepare for retirement?
9. What 'changes' may affect the older person's sexuality?
10. Identify the causes of erectile dysfunction and discuss how it may be treated.
11. What cultural pressures are placed on the older person's sexuality?

12. Differentiate between emotional disorders occurring before and after the age of sixty-five.
13. Clearly distinguish between senile dementia (of the Alzheimer's type), multi-infarct dementia, and reversible dementia.
14. How may confusion and disorientation be reduced in the older patient?
15. Describe how the depressed older person thinks, feels and acts. Outline nursing care of the severely depressed older patient.

Discussion topics

1. What opportunities are available in your community to help promote emotional and mental health in old age?
2. Do women ever retire?
3. "Nursing homes must be run by people with sexual problems – otherwise it would be difficult to explain the attempt to run them as mixed sex nunneries" (Alex Comfort, 1976). Discuss this statement.

Exercises

1. Visit a relative-carer for at least one day and:
   (a) identify basic demographic data (age, sex, marital status, education, employment, social security recipient?) concerning:
      i. the affected person; and
      ii. family carer.
   (b) describe the environment of the home in terms of:
      i. suitability for needs of the affected person;
      ii. security aspects.

(c) identify the problems of living for the:
   i. affected person;
   ii. carer/s;
   iii. community generally.

(d) describe the resources used by:
   i. the affected person;
   ii. family carer/s.

(e) identify any resources not used and try to establish why they aren't used.

2. View the film/video "Where's the key?" (BBC film) and identify which of the following areas caused difficulties for the sufferer of Alzheimer's disease and/or the relative-carer:
   - bathing
   - nutrition
   - elimination
   - mobility
   - memory
   - sleep
   - thinking
   - perception
   - emotions
   - social behaviour
   - communication

References

1. Crandall RC. Gerontology: a behavioural science approach. Reading, Massachusetts: Addison-Wesley Publishing Co. 1980.
2. Kart CS, Metress ES, Metress JF. Aging and health: biologic and social perspectives. Menlo Park, California: Addison-Wesley Publishing Co. 1978.
3. Ebersole P, Hess P. Toward healthy aging. St Louis: C.V. Mosby, 1985.
4. Erikson EH. Childhood and society. New York: Norton, 1964.
5. Dennis LB. Psychology of human behaviour for nurses. Philadelphia: W.B. Saunders, 1967.
6. Butler R. Why survive? Being old in America. In Kart CS, Metress ES, Metress JF. Aging and health. Menlo Park, California: Addison-Wesley Publishing Co. 1978.
7. Carnevali DL, Patrick M, eds. Nursing management for the elderly. Philadelphia: J.B. Lippincott Co. 1979.
8. Murray R, et al. The nursing process in later maturity. Englewood Cliffs, New Jersey: Prentice-Hall Inc. 1980.
9. Hamilton-Smith J. SPAN: First and second progress reports. Brotherhood of St Laurence, 1979 and 1981.
10. Division of Health Promotion. Getting on. Sydney: Health Commission of New South Wales, 1983.
11. Fox A. Foster grandparents. Growing Older 1972; 3(2): 10-11.

12. Landsbury R. Older workers and retirement. In Howe AL, ed. Towards an older Australia. University of Queensland Press, 1981.
13. Martin J, Doran A. Evidence concerning the relationship between health and retirement. Sociological Review Vol. 14, 1966.
14. Minkler M. Research on the health effects of retirement: an uncertain legacy. Journal of Health and Social Behaviour 1981; 22: 117-130.
15. Lansbury R. Older workers and retirement. In Howe AL, ed. Towards an older Australia. University of Queensland Press, 1981.
16. Morrison MH. Planning for income adequacy in retirement. The Gerontologist 1976; 16(6): 532-543.
17. Your money. Daily Telegraph 10 June, 1983.
18. McCallum J. Pre-retirement education programme. Work and People 1982; 8(3): 27-28.
19. Bowman K. Planning can prevent nightmare. The Australian 22 April, 1983.
20. Stubbs V. Preparation for retirement. Nursing Mirror 25 Sept. 1975.
21. Retirement. How to use your leisure time. Health Standard January 1978; 3-4.
22. Keating NC, Cole PW. What do I do with him 24 hours a day? Changes in the housewife role after retirement. The Gerontologist 1980; 20(1): 84-88.
23. Markley VJ. Sexuality and ageing. In Lion EM, ed. Human sexuality in nursing process. New York: John Wiley & Sons.
24. Wright D. Sex and the elderly. Nursing Mirror 1985; 161(5): 18-19.
25. Byers JP. Sexuality and the elderly. Geriatric Nursing Sept/Oct 1983; 293-297.
26. Eliopoulos C. Geriatric nursing. London: Harper & Row, 1979.
27. Friedeman JS. Factors influencing sexual expression in ageing persons: a review of the literature. Journal of Psychiatric Nursing and Mental Health Services 1978; July: 34-36.
28. Daines B, Holdsworth V. Time for talking. Nursing Mirror 7 Oct 1981; 20-21.
29. Merlin M. Sexual behaviour in the elderly. Paper presented at the NSW College of Nursing, Sydney, 1977.
30. Puksta NS. All about sex . . . after a coronary. American Journal of Nursing 1977; April: 602-612.
31. Daines B, Holdsworth AV. Impotence. Nursing Times 5 May, 1982; 763-765.
32. Griggs W. Sex and the elderly. American Journal of Nursing 1978; August: 1352-1354.
33. Pitt B. Psychogeriatrics: an introduction to the psychiatry of old age. Edinburgh: Churchill Livingstone, 1982.
34. Butler RN, Lewis MI. Ageing and mental health. Positive psychological and biomedical approaches. St Louis: C.V. Mosby, 1982.
35. Merlin M. Lectures to psychiatric nurse educators. Unpublished papers, 1980.
36. Verwoerdt A. Clinical geropsychiatry. Baltimore: Williams & Wilkins, 1981.
37. Henderson AS. The coming epidemic of dementia. Canberra: The Australian National University, 1984.
38. Brodaty H, et al, eds. Dementia: a handbook for the sufferer, and those caring for and helping the person with Alzheimer's disease and other related disorders. Sydney: Regency Press, 1983.
39. Wurtman RJ. Alzheimer's disease. Scientific American June, 1985; 48-56.
40. Broe GA. What is dementia? Unpublished paper, Sydney, 1984.
41. Summers WK, Majovski LV, Marsh GM, Tachiki K, Kling A. Oral tetrahydroaminoacridine in long-term treatment of senile dementia, Alzheimer's type. The New England Journal of Medicine 1986; 315(20): 1241-1245.
42. Sainsbury MJ. Key to psychiatry. Sydney: Australian & New Zealand Book Co. 1980.

43. Mace NL, Rabins PV. The 36-hour day. Baltimore: The Johns Hopkins University Press, 1981.
44. Gilleard CJ. Living with dementia. Community care of the elderly mentally infirm. Philadelphia: The Charles Press, 1984.
45. Williams S. The Lidcombe hospital dementia clinic. A new approach to managing dementia. Unpublished paper, Sydney.
46. American Psychiatric Association. Diagnostic and statistical manual of mental disorders. Washington DC: APA, 1980.
47. Steele D, Feldman RG. Diagnosing dementia and its treatable causes. Geriatrics 1979; March: 79-88.
48. Yesage J. Dementia: differential diagnosis and treatment. Geriatrics 1979; Sept: 51-59.
49. Stoulemire A, Thompson TL. Recognising and treating dementia. Geriatrics 1981; 36(10): 112-120.
50. Prochachazka Z, Henschke P, Skinner E, Last P. Memory loss and confusion. Dementia: a guide for caring people. South Australian Health Commission, 1983.
51. Stuart GW, Sundeen SJ. Principles and practice of psychiatric nursing. St Louis: C.V. Mosby, 1979.
52. Taylor CM. Essentials of psychiatric nursing. St Louis: C.V. Mosby, 1982.
53. Robinson L. Psychiatric nursing as a human experience. Philadelphia: W.B. Saunders Co. 1983.
54. Whitehead T. Confusing states of confusion. Nursing Mirror 1978; Sept 21: 29-30.
55. Ebaugh FG. Management of common problems in geriatric medicine. Menlo Park, California: Addison-Wesley Publishing Co. 1981.
56. Libow LS, Sherman FT. The core of geriatric medicine. St Louis: C.V. Mosby, 1981.

Chapter 8

Common Physical Problems in Old Age

Objectives

To enable the reader to:

1. discuss the ways in which disease presentation in older persons differs from that in younger age groups;
2. appreciate the importance of thorough assessment in the older person;
3. describe the causes and management, in the older patient, of:
   (a) falls
   (b) insomnia
   (c) constipation
   (d) hypothermia
   (e) pressure sores
   (f) urinary incontinence.

The process of ageing proceeds at different rates in different individuals and in different systems of the same individual.[1,2] Pathological processes may also develop gradually. With these two processes going on simultaneously it is not always easy to say what is a normal process and what is a disease state. This confusion can occur with osteoporosis, atherosclerosis, and impairment of control of body temperature and maintenance of blood pressure.[3] With these few exceptions, the nurse should be able to appreciate that there is a clear distinction to be drawn between changes produced by the normal ageing process (see Chapter 2) and those directly attributable to disease.

Altered disease pattern in the older adult

All too easily it is assumed that any manifestation of disease will be the same whether the patient is young or elderly. The daily practice of geriatric medicine and nursing shows that this is not true. Most states of disease are, in fact, modified to some extent by old age.[1] In particular, the following features of disease pattern are noted in the elderly.

Multiple pathology

A study conducted at a large geriatric hospital in Sydney in the 1970s showed that, on autopsy, older patients had on average six discrete diseases.[4] Other studies have shown similar findings which together represent serious problems for the older patient. The assessment of an elderly patient must therefore include investigations for all possible risk factors, all conditions present in all systems, including physical, psychological and social problems, and their potential for interaction. Some of the more common problems appear in Table 8.1.

Table 8.1 Common Clinical and other Problems in the Elderly

• Osteoarthritis	• Dizziness
• Osteoporosis	• Depression
• Confusion	• Urinary urgency
• Urinary incontinence	• Chronic renal failure
• Constipation	• Living alone
• Congestive cardiac failure	• Transportation problems
• Cerebral thrombosis	• Inadequate heating and cooling
• Unstable gait	• Sleep disorders

Appropriate priority will need to be given to the investigation of each problem identified. Where it is unclear which problem is causing the particular symptoms which the older person presents with, it is important to treat one problem at a time and assess the results.

Altered prevalence of disease

There are some diseases which occur more commonly in the elderly and there are others which occur almost exclusively in the older age group. Diseases which are more common in the elderly include:

- cerebrovascular accidents
- prostatic disease
- Parkinson's disease
- Alzheimer's disease

Diseases occurring almost exclusively in the elderly include:

- osteoporosis
- Alzheimer's disease
- accidental hypothermia
- calcific mitral annulae disease
- polymyalgia rheumatica
- monoclonal gammopathy
- multiple myeloma

Other diseases occur at all ages but have special implications for the elderly person. These include:

- hypertension
- diabetes mellitus
- pneumonia
- depression
- pulmonary emboli
- urinary tract infections
- stroke
- osteoarthritis
- hypo- and hyperthyroidism

Atypical presentation of disease

Often the presentation of many illnesses in the elderly is atypical, thus increasing the number of potential diagnoses. Ham *et al*[4] suggest the following atypical presentations of illness:

- silent malignant disease
- painless myocardial infarction
- silent pulmonary embolism
- nondyspnoeic pulmonary oedema
- afebrile pneumonia
- the silent surgical abdomen

It is possible then to find the following in the older patient:

- an altered response to pain associated, for example, with myocardial infarction, pneumothorax, or acute abdomen;
- no temperature in, for example, pneumothorax and pyelonephritis;
- missing symptoms, for example, no angina on exertion in heart disease, and no breathlessness on exertion in congestive cardiac failure.

Physical disorders resulting in mental impairment

Almost any physical disorder and psychosocial event has the potential to produce acute confusion in the older person (see Chapter 7).

Additional complications

Illness in the elderly may lead to a number of complications which are of significance for nursing care. These include:

- pressure sores
- contractures
- deep-venous thrombosis
- chest infection
- urinary tract infection

Non-specific presentations

Many illnesses which are well-defined in younger adults may present in very subtle and unexpected ways in the older adult.[4] Symptoms may include:

- lassitude
- tiredness
- anorexia
- loss of weight
- confusion
- anxiety
- tremor
- dizziness
- fatigue

Failure to diagnose possibly treatable, reversible diseases because of the vagueness of their presentation may have significant or even fatal consequences for the older adult.

Mixture of psychological, social and physical factors

Attempts to treat physical illness in isolation from psychological makeup and the social circumstances of the older patient will not be successful. One of the great challenges of geriatric medicine and nursing is to obtain all the relevant data about the client's physical and psychological status.

Unreporting of illness

Old people soon realise that complaining about symptoms tends to alienate others, so many old people tend to tolerate physical and psychological problems rather than attend to them. Still others assume too readily that their problems are an inevitable consequence of increasing age. Other possible reasons for non-complaint include denial, fear of what might be found, and the embarrassment associated with mental illness.

In a classic study by Anderson[4] during the 1950s in Scotland, a large number of untreated diseases were found among the elderly, despite free care. But if the older person did not complain specifically of being unwell, then no investigations were undertaken by the patient's doctor; or it was too readily accepted by the doctor that where problems were complained of they were related to 'old age'. Unfortunately, the older person was too often seen in a hospital at an advanced stage and with considerable disability.

Efforts to counteract this phenomenon must be made by health professionals and the public generally by educating older clients, their families, doctors and society.

Accumulation of conditions

There are many chronic, degenerative or disabling conditions which people accumulate in the course of their lives and which once acquired are never lost.[3] These may include:

- osteoarthritis
- disc degeneration and spondylosis
- foot deformities
- chronic lung diseases
- arterial disease
- cerebral ischaemia
- peripheral vascular disease
- chronic psychiatric disorders

The effect of iatrogenic disability

The patient with multiple problems is at a high risk of being placed on multiple drugs, and the elderly, therefore, are at special risk of drug-induced illness.[3,4] The reader is referred to Chapter 9 for the reasons why the elderly do not tolerate drugs well. Iatrogenic disability may be related to:

- physiological changes associated with normal ageing changes;
- the result of drugs;
- multiple prescribing;
- impaired compliance;
- pharmacodynamic changes which make the older person much more sensitive to many drugs;
- too many doctors becoming involved in treatment.

Iatrogenic illness can also be induced by hospitalisation and institutionalisation or by over-vigorous physical therapy. Remember, too, that psychological and behavioural problems can be iatrogenic illnesses. Mental confusion is a classic example.

Illness caused by sudden change

Balance is tipped more easily towards breakdown by an acute medical problem or a sudden change in the older person's social support system. An acute infection, physical trauma, or drug effect may be enough to cause the older person to experience a sudden and severe physical or psychosocial breakdown. Similarly, the death of a spouse or moving from the usual living arrangements (say to a nursing home or to hospital) may cause the older adult to break down into illness.

Assessment of disease in the older adult

All these features of the altered disease pattern in the older adult indicate clearly the importance of a thorough and competent physical and psychosocial assessment. Unless the initial examination is thorough, some important aspects of the illness or disability may be missed, with possibly fatal results. The reader is referred to Chapter 6 for a description of nursing assessment of the older adult.

Common clinical problems in old age

For practical purposes, Brocklehurst and Hanley[3] propose that it is better to think of problems experienced by the older adult than to use diagnostic labels. The problems of particular significance for the elderly are those that reduce mobility and 'addle the brain'.[5] The latter will not receive attention here but some of them are dealt with in Chapter 7. The contents of any good geriatric medicine or nursing textbook will indicate clearly what the common clinical problems are.

Several authors have attempted to categorise the major physical and psychosocial problems experienced by the older adult. Cape[4] describes them as being:

- falling
- confusion
- incontinence
- impaired homeostasis
- iatrogenic disorders

Coni, Davison and Webster[4] have conceptualised the problems of the aged as being:

- intellectual failure
- instability/immobility
- incontinence

The following clinical problems may be placed within such frameworks.

Falls

The disruption in the older person's lifestyle caused by an accident is highly significant. Even seemingly minor falls cause the older person to be confined to home, bed or hospital for a few days or even longer. Bedrest in particular increases the risk of complications which may be even more dangerous than the original fall. Older individuals over seventy years of age are at particular risk.[2,6,7]

Causes of falls generally have been identified by Garrett[4] as:

- cardiovascular disorders
- musculoskeletal disorders
- metabolic disorders
- neurological disorders
- environmental factors
- iatrogenic factors

To these may be added the normal changes associated with ageing (e.g. altered posture with changed centre of gravity, decreased muscle strength, slowed reaction time, loss of visual acuity).

In Riffle's study,[7] falls in the home occurred more frequently in the lounge room, hall, bedroom and on the stairs and were found to be related to slippery surfaces, loose rugs, poor lighting, and defects in door steps, carpeting and household furnishings. Dizziness, sudden malaise or weakness, difficulty in walking, confusion, dementia, poor eyesight, alcohol consumption, chronic disease, fainting and drug consumption also contributed. In a study by Odetunde[8] of falls of older people in hospital, it was found that:

- men fell more frequently than women (see also Riffle[7]). However, other studies have found the reverse to be true (e.g. as reported in Ham *et al*[4]);
- most falls occurred when the hospital personnel density was highest (see also Riffle[7]). Other studies (e.g. Feist, in Ebersole and Hess[2]) report that most falls occurred between 6 pm and 9 pm and 9 am to 12 noon;
- most falls took place in the first few weeks after admission.

Falls in hospital are associated with the need to urinate or defecate and acute illness.[7] Odetunde[8] noted Parkinson's disease as the commonest diagnosis associated with falls, followed closely by cardiovascular disease and a history of previous falls. The picture was far more complex than this, however, as most of the fallers had a history of multiple diagnoses. To this list can be added epilepsy (from a variety of causes), drop-attacks, transient ischaemic attacks, postural hypotension, syncope, Stokes-Adams attack and intermittent cardiac arrhythmias.[3]

A significant reduction in the number of falls in hospitals may be achieved by:

- reviewing staff numbers at times when falls are more frequent;
- regular staff education on how to handle the older patient safely;
- safety checks of ward furniture and equipment;
- using appropriate beds and ward furniture that will not easily move or tip over;
- cleaning well and appropriately before floors are walked upon;
- removing unnecessary obstacles;
- answering the older patient's call for assistance quickly;
- never leaving the older patient unattended in the toilet or bathroom for long periods of time;
- use of Ambularm (Widder, 1985) to alert staff when patient tries to get out of bed;
- conducting your own research as to why falls occur where you work.

The reporting of falls is extremely important. In particular, the nurse should be alerted if the older patient complains of persistent pain or headaches. Any program designed to prevent falls in the older population will require education of the older person and his family as well. Such a program could consist of relaxation and an exercise routine. Obviously, treatment of the underlying cause will be undertaken initially.

Insomnia

Inability to sleep (or insomnia) is very common among the aged population. With increasing age there are characteristic changes in the pattern of sleep and its duration. These changes may be normal[2,4,6,9] or they may be due to illness and other causes.

Basically, sleep is divided into REM (rapid eye movement) sleep, during which dreams take place, and NREM (non-rapid eye movement) sleep which includes all the other stages of sleep.[4] REM sleep is a deep physiological state which produces loss of muscle tonus, irregular pulse and elevated blood pressure, and is necessary for good health.[10] REM and NREM sleep alternate throughout the night. With extreme old age there may be a slight reduction in REM sleep. With increasing age there is a reduction in the quantity of NREM sleep. These changes may be considered normal in the older adult and should be differentiated from insomnia related to other causes (see Table 8.2).

Management of insomnia

Drug management of insomnia might include the use of hypnotics or anxiolytic agents. Where possible, however, it is far more desirable to identify and ameliorate the cause of the insomnia.

Essential information to obtain when assessing the problem consists of a sleep history, medication review, daily activity pattern, and physical and psychosocial health status. Various sleep charts have been developed to help assess the older person's sleep behaviour while in hospital.

Principles of good management would include:

- regular activity and mild exercise to promote rest and relaxation;
- breathing exercises and relaxation techniques;
- urinal, bedpan or commode kept near at hand, especially at night;
- non-use of sedation unless absolutely necessary;
- checking all drugs for adverse reactions;
- relief of depression;
- environmental modification;

Table 8.2 Causes of Insomnia in Old Age

Physical	
• nocturnal micturition	• fever
• leg cramps	• hyperthyroidism
• pain	• effects of drugs
• cough	• dyspnoea
Psychological/psychiatric	
• nightmares	• anxiety
• worry	• dementia
• bereavement	• confusion
• depression	• alcoholism
Environmental	
• noises in the environment	
• condition of the mattress	
• room temperature changes	
• lighting	

- nutritional changes;
- avoiding naps;
- use of music to promote relaxation;
- planned educational program to inform the older person about aged sleep changes and their causes and possible management.

Constipation

The aged are known for their concern about their bowel function and often make their concerns known to health professionals involved in their care. One of the most frequent complaints is about constipation. Basically, this is a diminished frequency of bowel action that represents a change in bowel habits or pattern.[2] Prolonged periods with no bowel action result in the withdrawal of fluid from the faecal mass through the large bowel wall. The stool, therefore, becomes progressively harder and difficult to evacuate.[4]

'Normal' elimination, of course, varies from one old person to another, so it is important to elicit from the older person what has been their pattern of elimination over the years and compare these data with the present episode of constipation.

Problems associated with constipation need to be managed as quickly as possible. These include the formation of pouches or diverticuli in the colon wall, and increasing abdominal pressure creating hiatus hernias.[2] Table 8.3 provides a list of the causes of constipation in the elderly.

Table 8.3 Causes of Constipation in the Elderly

• overuse of laxatives • immobility • inadequate fluid intake • diminished muscle tone and motor function • postponement of defecation reflex • dementia • the effect of some drugs (e.g. iron, codeine derivatives, aluminium compounds, antacids, anticholinergics, antidepressants)	• insufficient dietary bulk • dependence on others for aid in defecation • blunting or loss of defecation reflex • depression • hypothyroidism and diabetes • cancer of the bowel, diverticulosis, cancer of the rectum, anal fissures, haemorrhoids

Faecal impaction (constipation) can actually present as diarrhoea, which can be quite misleading. Here the constipation acts like a ball valve that intermittently allows liquid stool from higher levels to leak around it. Digital examination of the older person will help to eliminate this possibility.

Management of constipation

The older person's history will include their elimination behaviour and the nurse should appreciate the frequency of occurrence of constipation in the older population. The nurse must understand constipation, its causes and management in the older adult. For most older people the addition of fibre to the diet will be all that is necessary. Exercise will help to stimulate the colon and bowel evacuation. Most older patients can be educated about the range of normal movements.[11] Where it is not possible to alter their situation very much, regular treatment with either purgatives, suppositories or enemas may be useful.[3]

Hypothermia

An elderly person is hypothermic when his deep (core) temperature falls below 35 °C measured rectally.[12] This condition often goes unrecognised because ordinary rectal and oral thermometers do not register below 35 °C, or because complications (e.g. myocardial infarction or cerebrovascular accident) may dominate the clinical picture.[4] Some older adults are unable to maintain deep body temperature above 35 °C because their circulation and heat preserving mechanisms do not react normally to cold. Causes of hypothermia in the elderly appear in Table 8.4.

Table 8.4 Causes of Hypothermia in Old Age

Environmental
- older person is in a cold environment for some time
- poor insulation of houses
- inadequate clothing
- inadequate heating
- high heating costs
- poverty
- substandard housing

Physical
- immobilisation
- drugs (e.g. phenothiazines, imipramine, salicylates, barbiturates)
- reduced metabolic rate in hypothyroidism
- effect of ageing itself
- effect of cardiovascular disease
- effect of cerebrovascular disease

Psychological/psychiatric
- defiant independence
- loss of interest in life
- depression

Hypothermia can usually be diagnosed by feeling the patient's body, but suspicion and initial findings can only be substantiated by using a low-level rectal thermometer. The range of clinical features are included in Table 8.5.

Table 8.5 Clinical Features of Hypothermia in the Elderly

- the body is cold to touch
- the skin is cold and waxy
- the face looks myxoedematous
- the muscles are rigid and reflexes are diminished
- the ECG may show a characteristic J wave
- oliguria is common
- respiration is slow
- shallow and Cheyne-Stokes breathing is not uncommon
- bradycardia
- pallor
- somatic tremor
- apathy, possible disorientation, hallucinations or paranoid features
- progressive decline of body temperature will produce coma and may lead to eventual death

Management of hypothermia

A word of caution first. The older adult may not always feel or complain of being cold, and they can be cold even in hot weather. Treatment of hypothermia is extremely urgent. This will include:

- slow warming by wrapping the patient in a warm blanket and ensuring that the environment is warm;

- administering hot drinks if the patient can tolerate them;
- cardiac monitoring to detect the occurrence of cardiac arrhythmias;
- maintenance of a clear airway;
- antibiotics to prevent chest infections.

Prevention of hypothermia in old age will require:

- concern about and intervention in the older adult's environment;
- adequate money for heating fuels;
- use of an electric blanket in winter and at other times as necessary;
- adequate home insulation.

Pressure sores

Pressure sores, decubitus ulcers and bedsores are terms used to describe the same phenomenon. Pressure sores form because the skin and underlying tissue ulcerate when sufficient pressure is applied continuously to various parts of the body. This pressure causes ischaemia and eventually tissue necrosis.[9] Elderly people are at particular risk because of their thin, atrophic skin and lack of subcutaneous fat. Predisposing factors include:

- immobility
- sensory, perceptual or motor dysfunctions which impair the patient's ability to perceive discomfort and react appropriately
- impaired mobility
- malnutrition
- incontinence
- anaemia
- diabetes
- dehydration
- oversedation
- thinness
- physical debility related to various illnesses, e.g. cancer

Tissue breakdown may be aggravated by:

- poor nursing care
- urine and faeces in the patient's bed
- food crumbs in the bed
- failure to turn the patient routinely
- incorrect lifting technique

Ham *et al*[4] describe the development of pressure sore formation as follows:

- An area of erythema forms.
- A break in the skin occurs but with incomplete penetration.
- This extends subcutaneously, then superficially or deeply, and ultimately down to the muscle and through to the bone.

Table 8.6 indicates those body areas which are particularly susceptible to pressure sore formation.

Table 8.6 Body Areas Particularly Susceptible to Pressure Sore Formation

• If the patient is lying on his back	– shoulders – elbows – lower back – buttocks – heels
• If the patient is lying on his stomach	– knees – shins – pelvis
• If the patient is lying on his side	– hips – ankle
• Other susceptible areas	– underside of the scrotum – underneath the breasts – the pinna of the ear

Prevention of sores

Prevention of pressure sores is quite simple in theory. Obviously, those older patients who are at risk should be identified and the various factors contributing to the formation of sores prevented. Various instruments have been developed to help in this task (see Norton *et al;*[13] Brocklehurst and Hanley;[3] Ham *et al*;[4] Vincent[14]).

Management of pressure sores

Interventions in pressure sore formation may be achieved by:

Removal of pressure – here the older patient will need to be turned at least two hourly. The patient should be nursed on a water bed or ripple mattress and protection of the heels and buttocks may be achieved by means of sheepskin booties and a fleece. The patient should be lifted and turned by at least two nurses.

Adequate diet – a diet high in protein, carbohydrates and vitamins will be necessary for the healing of the ulcer. Adequate hydration will also be important.

Skin maintenance – the skin should be kept clean and dry and washed only when necessary, but never rubbed. All areas of skin over bony prominences and subject to pressure should be gently kneaded each time the patient is turned and regular inspection of the skin is essential.

Dressings – there are a great many ways of dressing pressure sores (see Ebersole and Hess;[2] Hibbs;[15] Finnegan;[16] Vincent[14]). The latest substance – Debrisan – consists of granules which are placed into the penetrating sore; care must be taken firstly to remove all the old granules. All dressings must be done under sterile conditions.

Surgical debridement – this is done by the patient's doctor in an attempt to remove necrotic tissue and stimulate the formation of healthy granulation tissue.

Care of pressure areas is a vital part of total care and makes an essential contribution towards the physical and psychological comfort of the older patient.

Urinary incontinence

Urinary incontinence is the lack of voluntary control of the evacuation of urine.[9] It may be either transient or chronic. Wells[17] estimates that 10 per cent of community elderly in the United States and 14 per cent in Britain are incontinent; 55 per cent of the elderly living in nursing homes in the US and 59 per cent in Britain are incontinent. One would expect to find a similar picture in Australia.

Urinary incontinence is one of the most important presenting symptoms of illness in the elderly, together with falls, immobility and mental confusion.[3] Because incontinence is a symptom, it will require careful investigation in order to determine the underlying causes – and these are numerous (see Table 8.7). At the least, incontinence is inconvenient and embarrassing and may cause the older person to stay at home rather than go out. The inconvenience of protective clothing and other devices, and the odour caused, result in altered levels and patterns of activity. These outcomes may lead to social isolation, dependency, loss of self-esteem and even depression.[4]

Investigations

Investigation of bladder function will be a necessary prelude to treatment. This will include:

History of incontinence. A detailed history of the incontinence is essential, with particular reference to its type and duration and the older

Table 8.7 Causes of Urinary Incontinence in Old Age

Physical	
• faecal impaction	• prostatic enlargement
• weakness of supporting pelvic muscles	• cystole, rectole and uterine collapse
• urinary tract infection or irritation	• atrophic senile vaginitis and atrophic urethritis
• dehydration	• bladder disease
• the effect of drug treatment (e.g. diuretics, antidepressants, bronchodilators, anti-Parkinsonian agents)	• failing vision
	• impaired mobility
	• inappropriate clothing
Psychological/psychiatric	
• depression	• dementia
• attention-seeking behaviour	• anger
• an attempt to manipulate the environment	• aggression
	• confusion
• embarrassment at asking for help	• anxiety
	• emotional shock, as in bereavement
Environmental	
• availability, size and location of toilets	• lack of privacy
• unfamiliar environment	• cot sides on beds

person's sensation and attitude to it.[6] The use of an incontinence chart may be helpful here (see Carnevali and Patrick;[6] Demmerle and Bartol;[18] Linke[19]). Information gathered should include:

- nature of urine;
- frequency and quantity of urine;
- circumstances of the episode;
- patient's emotional reaction to the episode.

Clinical examination. A complete pelvic and rectal examination should be carried out, including inspection of the vulva, urethral orifice, vagina, prostate gland and perineum. The bladder should be percussed and palpated. A thorough neurological examination should follow.[9]

Investigations. These could include:

- urinalysis
- cystoscopy
- cystometry.

Management of incontinence

When there is sufficient understanding of the problem, and the problem is transient, then management basically involves:

- treating the cause;
- good nursing care and regular toileting;
- pelvic floor exercises;
- habit training;
- biofeedback.

Where the incontinence is established, management could include a range of interventions, depending on the cause:

- antibiotics
- oestrogen
- anticholinergics
- catheterisation
- surgery
- physiotherapy

In the majority of cases the intervention/s will control the incontinence. Occasionally, though, there will be some patients who will not respond to any treatment. These patients will be managed with pads, appliances, catheters and good nursing care.[3]

Summary

It is important for the nurse to recognise the difference between changes associated with the normal ageing process and those which indicate that disease is present. With these two processes occurring simultaneously, this will not always be easy to do. Disease in the older adult may present somewhat differently from that in younger adults. To make this distinction clear, eleven differences are noted. The importance of accurate assessment, then, cannot be too strongly emphasised. Common physical clinical problems in the elderly are falls, insomnia, constipation, hypothermia, pressure sores and urinary incontinence.

Questions

1. Why is it so important to distinguish clearly between normal ageing changes and those related to disease?
2. In what specific ways does the pattern of disease differ in older patients compared with that in younger adults?
3. List six common clinical problems which occur in old age.
4. Why is a thorough assessment so important in the older patient?

5. Discuss falls as a clinical problem in old age under the following headings:
   (a) significance
   (b) causes
   (c) where they occur and under what circumstances
   (d) management and prevention.
6. What is insomnia? Why does it occur in the older adult? How is it managed?
7. How significant is constipation in the elderly? What complications can arise? What are its causes? Of what significance is faecal incontinence? How may constipation be managed?
8. When is an older person hypothermic? What are the causes of hypothermia? How may it be diagnosed? How may it be managed?
9. What are pressure sores? How do they form? How are they managed?
10. Describe urinary incontinence under the following headings:
   (a) definition
   (b) significance
   (c) complications
   (d) causes
   (e) investigations
   (f) management

Case study

Mrs Parkinson is a 77-year-old diabetic who lives on her own since her husband's death 12 months ago. She 'manages' on the pension. The community nurse has been asked by Mrs Parkinson's GP to visit because she has 'waterworks' problems, has fallen several times over the past month, and has increasing problems sleeping (waking several times during the night and difficulty getting back to sleep). Current medication is Melleril 25 mg b.d. and Noctec Syrup 500 mg Nocte.

As the community nurse talks with Mrs Parkinson it becomes obvious that she is extremely embarrassed about her 'waterworks' problems but is reluctant to discuss this. She puts it down to getting old. In discussing the situation with the daughter and Mrs Parkinson, the following facts are gathered:

1. Mrs Parkinson has a painful right hip which is shortened and externally rotated.
2. She is fragile and thin.
3. The 'waterworks' problems have been around for 12 months.
4. She refuses to go back and see her local GP.
5. The problems have restricted her getting out of the house.
6. She is very embarrassed by the 'waterworks' problems.
7. The daughter is becoming increasingly distressed about what to do and feels that her mother would be better off in a nursing home.

Task

1. Identify physical and psychological problems and potential problems.
2. For each actual problem, describe the possible physiological and psychological bases.
3. What diagnostic investigations may be necessary?
4. Outline the rationale for the management of actual problems.
5. What aids may be necessary and how might these be paid for?
6. Discuss the use of community resources and the involvement of family members and the client in her care.

References

1. Agate J. The practice of geriatrics. London: William Heinemann Medical Books, 1970.
2. Ebersole P, Hess P. Toward healthy ageing. St Louis: C.V. Mosby, 1985.
3. Brocklehurst JC, Hanley T. Geriatric medicine for students. Edinburgh: Churchill Livingstone, 1981.
4. Ham R, Holtzman JM, Marcy ML, Smith MR. Primary care geriatrics. Boston: John Wright, 1983.

5. Ford B. The elderly Australian. Harmondsworth, England: Penguin Books, 1979.
6. Carnevali DL, Patrick M. Nursing management for the elderly. Philadelphia: J.B. Lippincott Co. 1979.
7. Riffle KL. Falls: kinds, causes, and prevention. Geriatric Nursing Nov 1982; 165-169.
8. Odetunde Z. Fell walking. Nursing Mirror 24 Feb. 1982; 33-39.
9. Libow LS, Sherman FT. The core of geriatric medicine. St Louis: C.V. Mosby, 1981.
10. Lerner R. Sleep loss in the aged: implications for nursing practice. Journal of Gerontological Nursing 1982; 8(6): 323-326.
11. Goulston K. Rational management of constipation. Current Therapeutics July 1977; 43-44, 47-48.
12. Lye M, Kamal A. Old, cold and in danger of dying. Modern Geriatrics Nov. 1977; 40-43.
13. Norton C. Assessing incontinence. Nursing 1980; 1(18): 789.
14. Vincent GR. A survey uncovers some myths about pressure sores. The Australian Journal of Advanced Nursing 1984; 1(2): 22-37.
15. Hibbs P. Pressure sores: a system of prevention. Nursing Mirror 4 Aug. 1982; 25-29.
16. Finnegan D. Positive living or negative existence? Nursing Times March/April 1983; 53-59.
17. Wells T. Promoting urine control in older adults: scope of the problem. Geriatric Nursing Nov./Dec. 1980; 236-240.
18. Demmerle B, Bartol MA. Nursing care for the incontinent person. Geriatric Nursing Nov./Dec. 1980; 246-250.
19. Linke S. Behavioural analysis in the care of the elderly. Nursing Times 26 May 1982; 879-881.

Further reading

Belun R. A special recipe to banish constipation. Geriatric Nursing 1986; 6(4): 216-217.
Bloom MF. Dramatic decrease in decubitus ulcers. Geriatric Nursing 1986; 6(2): 84-87.
Hayter J. To nap or not to nap? Geriatric Nursing 1986; 6(2): 104-106.
Price M. Lecture notes for nurses. Sydney: Cumberland College of Health Sciences, 1984-85.
Schirmer MS. When sleep won't come. Journal of Gerontological Nursing 1983; 9(1): 16-21.
Thatcher RM. 98.6 °F – What is normal? Journal of Gerontological Nursing 1983; 9(1): 22-27.
Widder B. A new device to decrease falls. Geriatric Nursing 1986; 6(5): 287-288.

Chapter 9

Drug Therapy in the Elderly

Objectives

To enable the reader to:

1. identify factors related to drug misuse and medication errors among the aged;
2. describe physiological changes which may affect drug action in the elderly;
3. recognise adverse effects of specific drugs when used in the elderly;
4. discuss approaches to improving compliance of drug therapy in the elderly in the community setting;
5. describe common mistakes that occur in administration of medication to the aged in institutions.

The introduction of powerful modern medications has brought many problems for the elderly patient. Increased consumption, poor compliance, toxic and unwanted side effects, and changing physiology with ageing make the elderly more sensitive to the effects of drugs.

Increased consumption of drugs

The elderly are the fastest growing age group in our country and the largest consumers of health and pharmaceutical services. Although the pensioner age group makes up 9.2 per cent of Australia's population, it has been estimated that they probably consume about one-quarter of the prescribed drugs;[1] with some categories of drugs, such as psychotropics, 55 per cent are prescribed for the elderly age group.[2] The elderly are also heavy users of non-prescribed medication,[3,4] especially antacids and laxatives.

Antacids can affect the absorption of many drugs, potentiating some, such as quinidine, levodopa and sulphonamides; and inhibiting others such as digoxin, prednisolone, phenytoin, tetracyclines and many more.

Constipation is predominantly the result of immobility, poor dietary intake and drugs. Chemical bowel regulation can mask symptoms of underlying organic diseases or drug reactions. Bulk-forming agents or possibly a stool softener are preferable to the use of stimulant laxatives in the elderly.

How physiology of ageing affects drug responses

As a general rule, smaller doses of drugs are required to achieve the desired therapeutic results in the elderly. Changes in organ and tissue structure and function begin in the third and fourth decade and reach functional significance at a more advanced age.

Absorption

With ageing, extensive degenerative changes take place throughout the entire gastrointestinal tract; there are fewer absorbing cells, a reduced blood flow and reduced elasticity of musculature, especially in the colon. However, the rate and extent of drug absorption do not seem to be markedly affected by the ageing process.

Other drugs and diseases in the elderly may affect absorption more than ageing alone. Reduced absorption of iron, calcium and certain other essential vitamins and minerals has been demonstrated.[5] Drugs with a high first-pass effect, such as beta-blockers, may show a disproportionate increase in bioavailability in the elderly[6] and, as a result, lower doses of these drugs would be required. Concurrent administration of antacids or laxatives, many of which contain magnesium, aluminium or calcium, can adversely affect absorption of many drugs in the gastrointestinal tract.

Distribution

The decrease in weight, both of total body weight and of vital organs, with ageing is of important clinical significance.

The percentage of total body lipids increases from 15 per cent in young adult males to 36 per cent by the age of seventy-five (from 33 per cent to 45 per cent in women). As a result, the volume of distribution – and thus the duration of action – of lipid-soluble drugs such as chlorpromazine and diazepam increases in the elderly. Conversely, the volume of distribution of water-soluble drugs such as digoxin and gentamicin decreases and renders them potentially more toxic.

Cardiac output decreases by 30 per cent between twenty-five and sixty-five years of age and there is a corresponding decrease in blood flow to import target organs such as the liver, kidneys and brain. Drug distribution can be impaired as a result of the reduced blood flow. There may be a delay in the onset of drug action or a prolonged effect, as when removal to the site of metabolism is delayed.

Metabolism

Environmental factors such as smoking and diet may be equally or more important than ageing as a determinant of the variations between individuals in plasma levels of metabolised drugs.[6]

Reduced hepatic activity in older patients may manifest as a reduced first-pass effect, as with beta-blockers, or a prolonged half-life with drugs undergoing metabolism by Phase I processes such as oxidation or reduction (e.g. the long-acting benzodiazepines, nitrazepam and diazepam). Other benzodiazepines metabolised by Phase II processes such as glucouronidation and acetylation (e.g. oxazepam and lorazepam) appear to show no adverse effects on their metabolism with ageing.[6] These short-acting benzodiazepines that show no adverse effects in their metabolism with ageing are the preferred first choice for treatment if a sedative or anti-anxiety action is required.

Total serum protein concentration remains constant in the aged but albumin levels are on average 20 per cent lower than in young adults. Albumin binds and temporarily inactivates almost all drugs. A decrease in albumin results in an increase in 'free' (= active) drug and a greater drug effect. Drugs which are highly protein-bound, such as warfarin and phenytoin, will show this increase in free (active) drug to a greater extent in the older patient with reduced albumin. Use of more than one highly protein-bound drug will further complicate medical management of the elderly patient, with more competition for the reduced albumin.

Excretion

Age-related changes in renal function are the most significant factors in altered dosage requirements and drug effects in the elderly.

Renal function falls by 40-50 per cent by the age of sixty-five, regardless of any concurrent disease. Reduced kidney weight, number of nephrons and numbers of cells all decrease glomerular and tubular function.

In the elderly, drugs excreted primarily by the kidney will have a prolonged half-life and reduced clearance. This change is of great clinical significance for drugs such as the aminoglycoside antibiotics (gentamicin, neomycin, amikacin, etc.) and digoxin, which are all potentially toxic unless their dosages are reduced in older patients.

Target organ sensitivity

Changes in the sensitivity of receptor sites, especially in the brain, may result in abnormal drug effects in the elderly, effects that cannot be fully explained by the above physiological changes. A sedative such as nitrazepam may cause agitation and confusion despite 'normal' plasma levels; and phenothiazine drugs may cause parkinsonism-like symptoms and hypotension.

Deterioration of the autonomic nervous system with age is also likely to potentiate the hypotensive effect of centrally acting antihypertensive drugs such as methyldopa and clonidine.[7]

Toxic and unwanted side effects

Older people are more likely to suffer from more than one disease and consequently may be prescribed a number of different medications, in many cases by different doctors. Multiple drug therapy increases the possibilities of adverse drug reactions, patient confusion over instructions and also the likelihood of drug interactions, especially those due to additive pharmacological effects such as sedation and orthostatic hypotension.

The mechanisms of drug interaction are extremely complex and often poorly understood.

Typical manifestations of drug toxicity include 'inability to cope', recurrent falls, acute confusional state, generalised rigidity and urinary problems. The drugs most frequently implicated are the psychotropics, potent antihypertensives, diuretics, hypoglycaemic agents and digoxin.[8]

Sleep disturbances, agitation and depression are common problems for the elderly. Psychotropic drugs, namely hypnotics, tranquillisers and antidepressants, are commonly prescribed for the problems mentioned. They should be used cautiously as they are notorious for inducing mental fuzziness and confusion in older adults. As a group the psychotropic drugs are highly lipid-soluble and protein-bound with an affinity for various body tissues such as heart, brain and adipose tissue. Age-related neuronal loss and physiological changes have a significant effect on their action. Common adverse effects include sedation, anticholinergic effects, extra-pyramidal symptoms, cardiovascular effects and tardive dyskinesia.

Elderly patients are especially susceptible to heart failure, high blood pressure and blood clot formation in peripheral and cerebral vessels. Age-related changes in renal function, metabolic rates, absorption and distribution can lead to toxic effects and adverse reactions to the drugs used to treat these disorders. For example, lower doses of digoxin are needed in the elderly because of their reduced body water and reduced albumin. Renal impairment and hypokalaemia predispose to digoxin toxicity as does concurrent administration of other cardiac drugs, such as quinidine, verapamil, amiodarone, diltiazem and nifedipine; and both thiazide and loop diuretics.

The main side effects of beta-blockers in the elderly are peripheral coldness and worsening of peripheral vascular disease and, more rarely, disturbance of glucose metabolism and excessive fatigue. They should be avoided in patients with obstructive airways disease. There may be some advantage in using cardio-selective and longer-acting preparations to minimise side effects and simplify drug taking.

Diuretic agents are some of the most commonly prescribed drugs in the elderly. Problems often encountered with them are hypokalaemia, interference with glucose metabolism (may unmask latent diabetes mellitus) and increased uric acid retention (may precipitate an attack of gout).[7] Glucose tolerance deteriorates progressively with advancing age, so glucose intolerance in the elderly may be interpreted as part of the ageing process, a side effect of some drugs or true diabetes. Diabetic coma is a serious and often fatal complication of aggressive diuretic treatment of the aged.

Compliance in the community setting

As the largest consumers of drugs, the elderly have a high potential for misusing their medications. It has been reported that 85 per cent of patients aged seventy-five years and over are responsible for taking their own prescribed medications.[9] In addition, the percentage of patients who make errors in taking their medications ranges from 25 to 59 per cent.[10] Four major ways in which the elderly fail to take their medications correctly are underdosage, overdosage, taking old medication from old prescriptions and taking other people's tablets. Omission is the most common error.[11]

Poor compliance may be attributed to a range of different problems. These include lack of knowledge, multiple drugs, complex regimens, inability to see or hear well, memory loss, social isolation, financial barriers, and failure of health professionals to give adequate instruction.[12]

Research and interest in compliance has seen a variety of health professionals becoming involved. Various strategies to improve compliance have been promoted in the literature to individual clinicians in nursing, pharmacy and medicine.[13-15] An outline of some of the strategies recommended to date[14] is given in Table 9.1.

Table 9.1

Barrier to Compliance	**Method**
Hearing impairment	– Speak loudly and slowly.
	– Face the patient directly.
Impaired vision	– Label all written information with large letters using bold-face type.
	– Use a colour coding system or different shaped bottles for recognition by touching.
Memory loss	– Distribute patient package inserts to reinforce physician and pharmacist instructions and to be home 'reference guides'.
	– Repeat instructions.
	– Evaluate every patient's comprehension of drug instructions using non-threatening non-judgmental questions.
Dexterity problems	– Advise of the availability of non-childproof medication containers.
Complex drug regimen	– Put name and purpose of medication on containers.
	– Labelling should be simple, direct and understandable (e.g. Digoxin – heart pill)
	– Minimise number of times per day medication is required.
	– Eliminate unnecessary medications.
	– Use a patient profile system to record medications dispensed.
Social isolation	– Distribute medication calendars.
	– Involve available family members.
Lack of knowledge about drug use	– Provide specific detailed oral and written information about the drug regimen including purpose and type of medication prescribed, brand or generic name, dosage schedule, duration of therapy and whether drug should be taken continuously or symptomatically.
Diffidence towards health professionals	– Assure privacy in the practice setting. Provide older patients with time to ask questions.
Cost of drugs	– Substitute generic drugs or less costly alternatives.
	– Suggest non-drug alternatives.
	– Discourage the use of unnecessary non-prescription drugs.

Source: ED-MED Manual (Education about Medications). G. Higgins, P. Hawe, F. Everingham. Lidcombe Hospital, Sydney, 1987.

Some of the strategies in Table 9.1 can be incorporated into a patient education program to enhance compliance. Pharmacists should be utilised to provide large-type labels with clear and unambiguous directions, medication calendars, preloaded multicompartment containers and medication cards where appropriate. Medication cards carried by patients, detailing patient name, address, allergies, medication name (generic and brand), strength, dose and use are very popular with patients and doctors.[12]

Compliance in the hospital setting

Polypharmacy, that is, the concomitant use of several drugs,[16] thrives among many elderly patients, especially those in institutions. It includes duplication of drug classes and unrecognised side effects being treated with more drugs. The contribution of a consultant pharmacist to minimise polypharmacy and related problems in the long-term care facility has been shown to reduce the average number of drugs from 7.2 to 4.8 over a year.[16]

Many errors can be made in a ward situation. Patients with severe dementia may not be able to identify themselves and nurses may not always be familiar with the patients under their care. Photographs on patients' beds and with patient treatment sheets, as well as name bracelets, make identification of patients easier and more reliable.

Discrepancies in drug administration also occur due to staff error. The error rate can vary from 32 to 64 per cent.[17] Traditional medication errors of wrong dose, wrong tablet, wrong time and wrong patient can be minimised by using a unit-of-use medication system. A unit-of-use pack is a package unit containing sufficient doses of a preparation for a course of treatment, e.g. a week's supply of antibiotics or a month's supply of a diuretic. The package is labelled with all the information needed to identify that preparation fully. The package can also be labelled for a specific patient for a specific time, reducing potential errors even more. The main benefits of a unit dose system are the reduction in medication errors, significant savings in nursing time, drug use control and reduction in drug wastage.[17,18]

Conclusion

Medication may be used appropriately and judiciously to produce significant improvement or recovery and thus make life more meaningful and pleasant for the ageing population. Changing physiology and special needs should be carefully considered, however, before any medications are used.

Before new drugs are prescribed the doctor should thoroughly review all medication the aged patient is currently taking. This includes all prescribed as well as all purchased medication. It is possible that the 'illness' may be an adverse drug reaction and stopping the drug may be more beneficial to the older person than starting others.

Non-compliance with medication regimens is a well-documented and major health problem for our ageing population. All health professionals are involved at some phase of compliance management and each has an important role to play in using effective strategies to encourage compliance in clinical practice, in the community and in the institutionalised setting.

Questions

1. What are the major mistakes made by the older person in taking medication?
2. List and briefly describe the specific physiological changes that occur in old age. How do these affect drug action in the elderly?
3. Describe the effects of altered physiology in old age on the action of the following:
   (a) psychotropic agents
   (b) digoxin
   (c) diuretics
   (d) gentamicin
   (e) beta-blockers
4. Discuss the possible actions which could help to reduce errors in medication administration in the older population in:
   (a) the hospital setting
   (b) the community setting

References

1. Wynne RD, Heller F. Drug overuse among the elderly: a growing problem. Perspectives on Ageing 1973; 11(1): 15-18.
2. Chapman S. Psychotropic drug use in the elderly. Medical Journal of Australia 1976; 2: 62-64.

3. Bush PJ. Who's using non-prescribed medicine? Medical Care 1976; 14: 1014-1023.
4. Levine P. Abuse of prescription and non-prescription drugs by older citizens reported rising. Retirement Living 1978; 18: 49-53.
5. Shaw PG. Pitfalls in geriatric prescribing. Current Therapeutics Oct. 1981: 45-49.
6. Triggs EJ. Paediatric and geriatric clinical pharmacy. 1982; 4(1): 6-10. Canberra: Pharmaceutical Society of Australia.
7. Martin A. Problems in geriatric medicine. Great Britain: Adis Press, 1981.
8. Gibian T. Drug therapy in the elderly. Unpublished paper presented at Lidcombe Hospital, Sydney, 1984.
9. Law R, Chalmers C. Medicine and elderly people: a general practice survey. British Medical Journal 1976; 1: 565-568.
10. Stewart RB, Cluff LE. A review of medication errors and compliance in ambulant patients. Clinical Pharmacology and Therapeutics 1972; 13: 463-468.
11. MacDonald ET, MacDonald JB, Phoenix M. Improving drug compliance after hospital discharge. British Medical Journal 1977; 2: 618-621.
12. Higgins G, Hawe P, Everingham F. ED-MED Manual (Education about Medications). Sydney: Lidcombe Hospital, 1987.
13. De Berry P, Jefferies LP, Light MR. Teaching cardiac patients to manage medications. American Journal of Nursing 1974; 75: 2191-2193.
14. Lipton HL. The graying of America: implications for the pharmacist. American Journal of Hospital Pharmacy 1982; 39: 131-135.
15. Haynes RB, Sackett DL, Taylor DW. How to detect and manage low patient compliance in chronic illness. Geriatrics 1980; 35: 91-97.
16. Vestal RE, ed. Drug treatment in the elderly. Sydney: Adis Health Press, 1984.
17. Miller B. The rationale of unit dose drug distribution systems. Australian Journal of Pharmacy April 1977: 232-235.
18. Goodman M, Woodbridge M. The effectiveness of a unit-of-use drug distribution system. Australian Journal of Hospital Pharmacy 1979; 9(1): 33-36.

Further reading

Drug treatment in old age: a seminar. Current Therapeutics Oct. 1983.

Rowe JW, Besdine RW. Drug therapy. In Rowe JW, Besdine RW. Health and disease in old age. Boston: Little, Brown & Co. 1982.

Chapter 10

Rehabilitation: An Interdisciplinary Approach

Objectives
To enable the reader to:
1. define rehabilitation and its philosophy;
2. discuss the rehabilitation process;
3. explore the concept of the team approach in rehabilitation;
4. define the role of the nurse in rehabilitation;
5. identify the range of rehabilitation services and have an appreciation of the resources available to facilitate independence;
6. describe the issues facing the older person in society. Identify how rehabilitation workers can meet the challenge of these issues.

The word 'rehabilitation' is derived from 'rehabilitare' meaning ' to restore to a former capacity' or, more specifically, 'to restore to a condition of health or useful and constructive activity'.[1]

It is difficult to determine exactly when the concept of rehabilitation evolved, but history records the belief of several western and near eastern civilisations in the restorative powers of spas, massage and exercise in convalescence from illness and battle. These include the Egyptians, Greeks, Romans and Arabs. Similarly, eastern civilisations have advocated the use of massage, meditation and herbs to restore health throughout their recorded history, considering them important enough to incorporate into cultural rituals.

Influence of nursing on the concept of rehabilitation

Probably no other discipline has influenced the development of a concept and philosophy of rehabilitation quite as strongly as nursing, and the reasons for this are primarily historical.

Nursing emerged as a recognised health discipline during the 19th century, the need for a 'people-orientated health service' being evident to both society and governments. It differed from medicine in two basic principles: it was not cure-based, and fundamental to nursing was the belief that 'only nature can cure'. Thus, historically, the basic tenets of nursing have been concerned with 'providing an environment in which nature can cure'.[2]

Essentially, nursing has maintained this belief, which is interpreted as being functionally restorative and holistic in orientation. It is not surprising, therefore, that the fundamental elements of a concept and philosophy of rehabilitation have been significantly influenced by the basic tenets of nursing. These are:

- Advocacy on the individual's behalf.[2,3] This is considered to be of such importance that it is incorporated into professional codes, e.g. International Council of Nurses, and the Royal Australian Nursing Federation Standards of Professional Practice.
- Service based on humanism.[1,3,4] This tenet is strongly aligned to advocacy and incorporates the notions of:
  - equality in the distribution of power in the nurse/individual relationship;[5-8]
  - holistically oriented service which incorporates the notion that the person's total environment is considered in relation to his past and present experiences and his future expectations (a personal interpretation);
  - the individual's right to self-determination, which includes the right to take risks as well as to make decisions.
- Continuity of service. This implies that interventions occur as planned, and to the standard required to achieve desired goals.

In action, these fundamental principles of nursing have significantly influenced the following events:

- the humanising of services to the psychiatrically ill and the development of formal systems of nursing rehabilitation from the 1850s;[4]
- the humanising and rehabilitation of female prisoners from the 1850s, primarily as a result of the efforts of the Sisters of Charity;

- the management of children who were victims of poliomyelitis from 1900 onwards, primarily through the efforts of Elizabeth Kenny;[9]
- humanistic services to the non-institutionalised aged, disabled and disadvantaged, primarily through the efforts of the Sydney Home Nursing Service, from 1900 onwards;
- the development of child and maternal health services through the efforts of midwives in private practice.[10]

These initiatives have helped to shape the contemporary concepts and philosophy of rehabilitation.

Concept of rehabilitation today

The concepts of rehabilitation today are educative in orientation, and philosophically aligned to the notion of individuals assuming responsibility for themselves by moving towards self-care models. These concepts embody an existential bias and move away from dependency and institutional models. Recent initiatives in health have demonstrated this trend, e.g. the Macleay and Richmond Reports of 1983. It is from these contemporary notions of rehabilitation that the process of rehabilitation has evolved.

The process of rehabilitation

In the preface of his book *Eggshells and Tea-leaves: Memories of an Ordinary Man*, Don Willis, aged 65 years, thanks the nurses and occupational therapists of the hospitals he attended for initially suggesting he "should try his hand at writing something – no matter what; my wife and family who kept me hard at it and refused to allow any slacking". A series of strokes had left him extensively paralysed and with impaired speech.

Don Willis was an exceptional person, undefeated by devastating odds. His book demonstrates that stroke-affected people who are determined to get better always do better in the long run by cutting across the neurological book of rules.

Morale is a vital factor in recovery and it is unique for each person. Negative reactions associated with a physical disability might include anger, feelings of injustice, futility, depression and a sense of hopelessness. Even in the presence of such negative feelings there is the sheer tenacity to hold onto life, a preference to be alive rather than dead. The factors that contribute to high morale are again unique to each individual. The art of rehabilitation is to capitalise on these factors.

The rehabilitation process is specific to the situation and centres on the individual. Its essence embodies psychological, social and biological forces. The process includes:

- the reformation of self, and physical, psychological and social changes;
- expectations of the self and the future;
- time factors;
- mood states.

The reformation of the self deals with body image, perceptions, and the loss of status roles in the community. Physical aspects include body image changes, altered perceptions, loss of ability to perform tasks, and decreased mobility. Psychological changes encompass anger, frustration, grief, loss of self-esteem, and depression. Social changes include limited social contacts, loss of previous social activities, role and financial changes.

Past personality development, life experiences, education, social relationships and the extent of support networks will shape the motivation and expectations of the self in relation to present and future activities and interactions. Time factors are important for the aged person, for improvements may take a number of years to achieve; people who have had a stroke may not notice improvements until many years after the initial event. Throughout this process the aged person will move from moods related to low self-esteem to a restored self-image; optimism and a level of acceptance will develop. Following a crisis, the individual passes from the known external world, through internalisation of the experience and the rehabilitation process, to a state of reflection and finally adaptation.

As with any life crisis, some people do not progress to the stage of acceptance or adaptation to their disability. The aged may have many problems to cope with and the rehabilitation process needs to be realistic, goal-oriented, holistic and flexible. To make small changes in a person's lifestyle is a major achievement.

The key issues in the rehabilitation process are:

- it is done *by* the individual, not *to* the individual;
- it is a personal, biological and social development.

The team approach to rehabilitation

Much has been written about the value of the team approach in rehabilitation and its contribution to the overall aim of returning individuals to the community with 'maximum independence as quickly as possible'. The word 'team' is a misused term for any group of people who meet periodically. It gives the impression that important business is taking place and that there is a high quality of interaction (Fig. 10.1).

Figure 10.1 Is this a team?

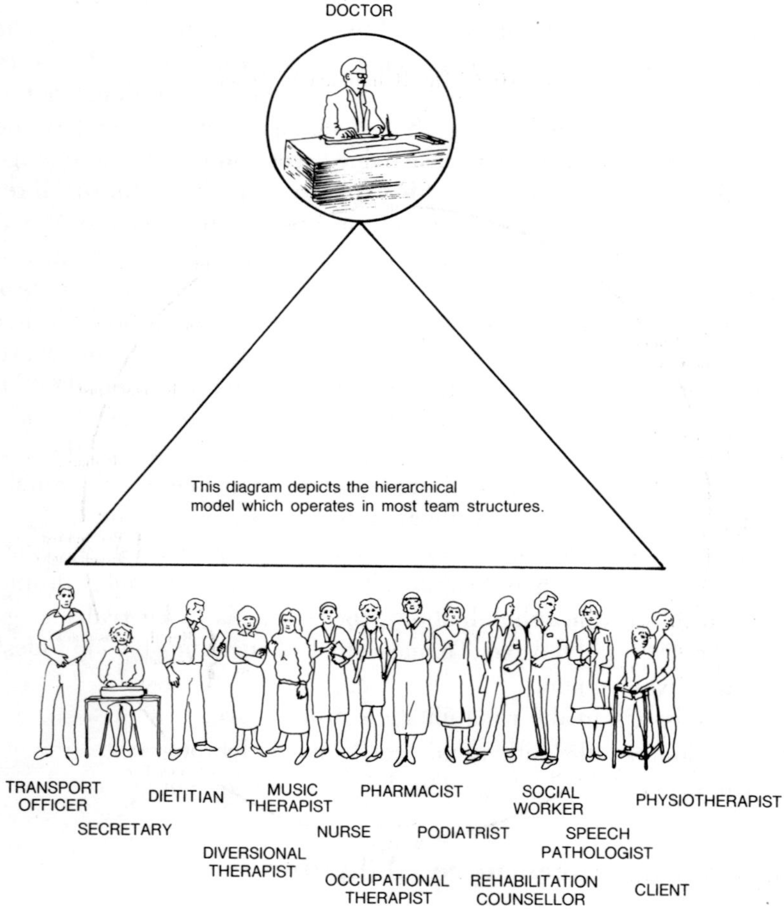

This diagram depicts the hierarchical model which operates in most team structures.

The word 'team' should describe the quite specific way a group of people work together. The ideal health care team is the interdisciplinary one where members of different disciplines are involved in formal and informal ways to provide an optimum service (see Fig. 10.2). Melvin[11] described the differences between 'multidisciplinary' and 'interdisciplinary', describing the first as 'activities involving the efforts of individuals from several disciplines. Their efforts are discipline-oriented although they operate in a multidisciplinary setting. Each member need only know the skills necessary for the practice of his/her own profession'.

Figure 10.2 The Rehabilitation Team

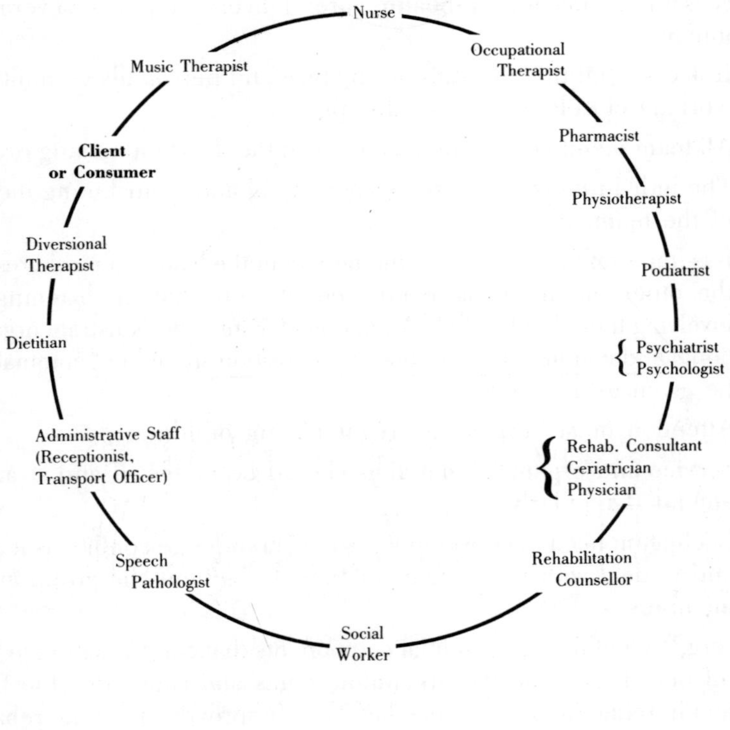

A rehabilitation team may consist of some or all of the above.

'Interdisciplinary' also refers to activities directed towards a common aim by individuals representing different disciplines. However, members have the added responsibility of group effort which 'requires the skills necessary for effective group interaction and the knowledge about how to transfer integrated group activities into a result which is greater than the sum of the activities of each individual member. The activity of an interdisciplinary team is synergistic, producing more than each could accomplish individually and separately'. A team operating at an optimum level, in conjunction with the individual (client) and family identifies realistic group aims, sets priorities, co-ordinates treatments, educational and counselling sessions, and plans for the discharge needs of the individual and family at an early stage of intervention. When the team is interacting at this optimum level both team members and individuals/families benefit. At this level of co-operation members can be seen to act as a resource/support network for each other and the client group. Ongoing learning takes place through the sharing of skills. The organisational aims of the service should be client-centred and thereby accountable to the local community.

Successful teamwork in health care delivery requires several key components:

- It is essential that the staff are mature and personally committed to working closely with other disciplines.
- All team members function as peers in the decision-making process.
- The individual/family is seen as an equal and contributing member of the team.
- It is important to ensure that the person in the leadership role respects the other members, as evidenced by consultation, listening and involving them in planning. A team leader must demonstrate organisational and communication skills. This position should not automatically be given to a doctor.
- Attention must be given to regular team building.
- Service and organisational aims should be reviewed and strategies amended regularly.
- Each team needs to develop ways to acknowledge conflict as it arises and to deal with it in a manner that strengthens the group and its members.

Rothberg,[12] identifies ten essential components that contribute to the formation of interdisciplinary rehabilitation teams and states that the future direction in rehabilitation practice lies in the improvement of the rehabilitation team, so that it becomes interdisciplinary rather than just multidisciplinary.

The rehabilitation team can consist of a number of health professionals. Membership and size will depend on the focus of the team, e.g. day hospital team, nursing home team, assessment team, community rehabilitation team, etc.

The role of the nurse in rehabilitation

> Nurses are rehabilitation par excellence and might have coined the phrase and described the process had they been more thoroughly educated, more analytical, and more aware of their potential role in society . . .[13]

Rehabilitation is a fundamental tenet on which nursing is based and, therefore, is viewed as a legitimate and integral part of the nurse's role, regardless of where they practise. This notion is supported by the accepted contemporary definition of nursing:

> The unique function of the nurse is to assist the individual, sick or well, in the performance of those activities contributing to health or its recovery that he would perform unaided if he had the necessary strength, will and knowledge. And to do this in such a way as to help him gain independence as rapidly as possible.[3]

This definition relates to basic nursing function and yet has a strong rehabilitation bias, as indeed it should. However, nurses practising in rehabilitation operate from a specialist role, so it is necessary to extend the basic definition in order to describe their function accurately.

> The role of the nurse is to enable the individual to achieve his maximum level of function, by assessment-based interventions implemented through a teaching mode aimed at independence in areas of mutually agreed human need, and evaluation of expected outcomes at regular intervals.

The above role description appears appropriate as it is consistent with the basic role definition and it incorporates the fundamental tenets of nursing: advocacy, humanism, holism, continuity and education. Concurrently it addresses the contemporary nursing ideas of:

- equality in the distribution of power in the nurse/individual relationship;
- the use of human needs criteria as a basis for assessment, e.g. existence needs, relatedness needs, growth needs;
- the need for research-based nursing practice;

- the use of scientific method in nursing practice, e.g. the nursing process;
- professional autonomy and concurrent accountability.

Major issues in rehabilitation nursing

Consistency in philosophy, objectives and practice

The role of the nurse practising in rehabilitation is a specialist one, which is expressed through the process of practice. Therefore, the fact that a nurse is employed within a community team, or in an institution, should not influence the method of practice, the philosophy behind it, nor the primary professional objectives. These should be consistent.

It is envisaged that in time the 'specialist' nature of the role of the rehabilitation nurse will, in effect, become the modus operandi of nurses generally. This will occur as nurses become better educated, more analytical, more secure in their concept of their value to society, and thus challenge the status quo on behalf of the community. Even though this may appear futuristic, it should be recalled that this has been a prime function of nursing since its inception, and it is only in recent times that nursing practice has become complacent and therefore unwilling to agitate on behalf of the community.

The need for research-based practice

In the past nurses have drawn primarily on medical knowledge for their body of professional knowledge, and hence their practice. The effects of this are evident to all nurses. It should be noted, however, that this link with the medical profession knowledge base has evolved over fairly recent times and it is in absolute conflict with the fundamentals on which nursing is based. Additionally, this situation is not particularly idiosyncratic to nursing, but is indeed true to all allied health professionals.

The need for practice-based research

Nurses practising in rehabilitation have a fundamental professional obligation to engage in practice-based research, for only in this way will the body of nursing knowledge increase. Research needs to be nursing and practice specific if it is to be incorporated into everyday practice.

The involvement of nurses in interdisciplinary team management

While nurses do have a discrete role in rehabilitation, they are in a position as members of interdisciplinary teams to overview the individual's total interactions with their environment. Nurses have an obligation to their colleagues to share, maintain and develop their unique skills, and in this way strengthen the knowledge base of the group.

The above issues are not rehabilitation specific, but are major issues confronting nursing generally.

Issues confronting the elderly in rehabilitation of particular concern to nurses can be identified as follows:

- slowed reaction times
- loss of sensory acuity
- decline in memory/delayed recall
- lowered endurance and energy
- altered sexual functioning
- powerlessness
- decreased status
- development of maladaptive behaviour patterns.

It is not inferred that all elderly people experience any, or all of the above, only that statistically the incidence to the above increases with age. Like all individuals, elderly people are unique and should be regarded as such. If nurses are to address these issues realistically they must operate from the individual's terms of reference.

The issues facing the older person in society

The issues facing the aged depend mainly on the perspective of those describing them. Rehabilitation workers experience certain constraints on the way they work which interfere with the potential that the aged person can see as a possibility for their own present and future.

The following is a list of constraints that may be operating on workers with the aged:

- definition or labels
- ageism
- the organisation
- education
- the health professional's personal values.

Definition

Why define the elderly as a problem? Should they be defined as a 'problem' or as a 'challenge'? Most elderly people are managing independently in their own homes. The people health workers see or hear about are in reality just a small minority of the aged population. Therefore, health workers are tending to define the elderly as a problem, based on a small sample. The aged are seen as a problem because society has not planned for this event. Instead, any planning efforts have been piecemeal and have tended to respond to crisis situations. At present there is an ageing bulge due to historical events and social changes which occurred throughout this century. These events included a falling birthrate, the immigration of young workers, family reunions and better living standards.

The alternative is to view working with the elderly as a challenge, where nurses and other health workers have an opportunity to work with an interesting group. The challenge in working with the elderly is finding the most appropriate service and being creative in finding new answers to new problems. The elderly are people who have had to adapt to great changes and upheavals in their lives.

Ageism

Ageism is a prejudice concerned with ignorance, deprivation of power and stereotyping. The most pervading constraint that impedes work with the elderly, with their family/friends, and with other health professionals is the widespread ageist views held by the wider society.

Health workers (including nurses) are culprits of ageism as they often collude with second-rate services that are provided for the elderly. Good examples of these are poor nursing homes, inadequate meals-on-wheels, unstimulating day care and inadequate respite care.

Often there exist health workers' negative feelings, which limit their involvement. One such feeling is that elderly people just require voluntary help or a practical problem solved and don't need a skilled person to look at their difficulty.

A common perspective often supported is that they are near the end of their lives, don't need much money to survive, should have planned their lives better, are too demanding, should be grateful for all that is done for them and can't participate fully in decision-making. At times they are perceived as disabled, frail, slightly demented, dependent. They are inarticulate, poor, powerless and without a future; or, alternatively, perceived as well off, powerful, scheming to get out of the assets test, or just too pushy.

Workers have to realise that many difficulties faced by the elderly are issues of poor housing, inadequate income security, high health costs and inaccessibility to a range of recreation options. They need to take a broader view of the elderly that encompasses health promotion and illness prevention. When this is achieved there will be more assertive and vociferous health workers who are prepared to advocate on behalf of the elderly.

The existing system provides a 'sick' dependent medical model which could bias health professionals' work with the elderly.

Often ageism is so subtle that it is easy to go along with decisions without realising how many of them are based on ageist assumptions. In rehabilitation, health workers are in contact with many professionals and agencies and are sometimes faced with other people's low expectations of the elderly. Often other professionals put pressure on the elderly to convince them that they can't cope any more. Often health professionals feel so responsible that they can't leave the decision and the accompanying risks with the elderly person.

Another source of pressure on the elderly and health workers emanates from the families or concerned others. It is necessary to weigh comments and criticisms, while maintaining the role of advocacy for the elderly person.

Even the elderly have internalised the stereotypes to such an extent that health professionals could easily reinforce their low expectations and feelings of worthlessness. The practice is questionable whereby low expectations are condoned in the face of inadequate resources. In this situation some workers limit the options they offer the elderly and accept the first rejection by the consumer. Positive discrimination may be essential for people who are so disadvantaged. They require a lot of time and encouragement. In some instances intensive work is required before the individual can become aware of options.

The organisation

By its very structure, the organisation can be a major source of frustration. Bureaucracies are not known for their flexibility or creativity.

Few organisations appear to have formal policies on services to the elderly. They may have broad objectives but many may be informal or relate to broader services than those specific to the elderly. What happens most often is that objectives are formulated within the agency to give guidelines on how to proceed.

The organisation may try to sell the line that it is quantity, economics and acute care that count. In the face of this, workers often feel powerless to even consider the elderly person at the end of the line.

The low status of workers in the organisation makes it easy to accept powerlessness as a *fait accompli*. This can lead to the organisation being excused for its view of the world and lack of responsibility. Workers can start to believe in the supreme importance of bed turnovers, or think that acute care is more important than chronic care, or that treatment is a higher priority than advocacy.

However, elderly people don't see health professionals as powerless. At times, workers function in isolation within agencies and forget the possible alliances that could be made with other professions and consumer agencies. The power of such consumer groups as the Combined Pensioners Association is often underestimated. If consumers are frightened or lack the confidence to articulate their situation then such groups as the Combined Pensioners Association may take up an issue for them.

Education

What the education curriculum of health professionals has lacked is emphasis on the importance of working with the elderly. This situation has led to a low status image for people working in this field. Health professions need to give value to working with the elderly. The initiative must come from the teaching institutions. Practitioners must put pressure on the education system for recognition of work in this field.

Health professional's personal values

Nursing has the capacity, by its very nature, to make nurses the most radical advocates for change. As primary health carers they are uniquely qualified for this task. It is necessary, however, to ask certain questions of oneself and to understand personal and professional expectations. Unless nurses are aware of their own values and the biases that arise from these values, they will be unable to intervene in the most positive manner. If nurses are meeting their own needs by fulfilling a charitable or compassionate side of their nature, they may have a limited view of their role. Nurses must question what personal/professional goals are being satisfied in their work with the elderly.

Rehabilitation services and resources available to facilitate independence

The range of rehabilitation facilities varies across the State as each Health Department Region has developed services to meet local needs. Some health regions have developed a more integrated area service than others, with close liaison between the various health department components and a close working relationship with services provided by the Local Authority and other State and non-government sectors.

While the facility may vary, the rehabilitation process remains the same. This process has been conceptualised in Figure 10.3. The reader will notice that the steps are not unlike those involved in the nursing process.

Figure 10.3 The Steps involved in the Client's Rehabilitation

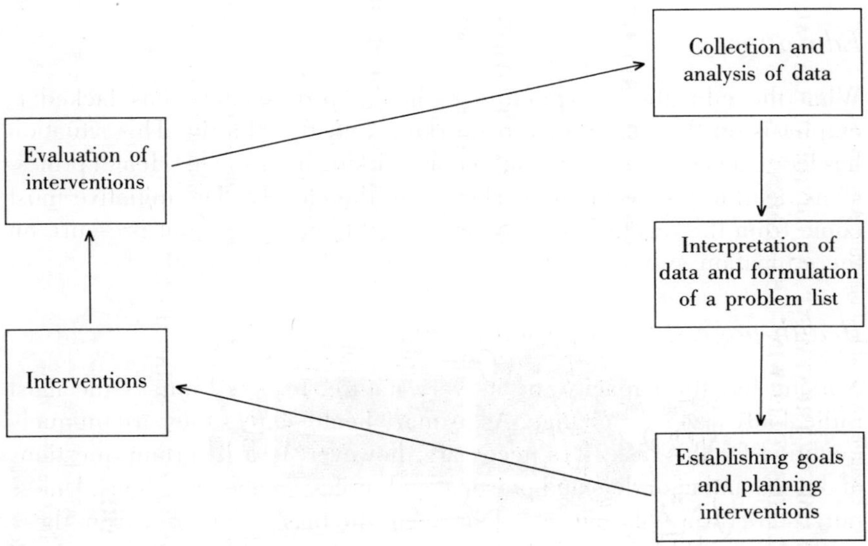

Depending on the level of dysfunction/disability and aims of treatment, an individual may attend one or more facilities following assessment (see Figs 10.4 and 10.5). The time allocated to this process varies with the complexity of the issues identified.

Institution-based services

Rehabilitation Department. Provides a consultative service to all hospital inpatients at request of admitting doctor and has a treatment area for use by inpatients and outpatients.

Rehabilitation Unit. Offers specially designed ward facilities which often include self-care component. Has appropriate treatment areas for inpatients and outpatients.

Figure 10.4 Facilities Available Following Assessment

DEPENDING UPON LEVEL OF DISABILITY AND AIMS OF TREATMENT AN INDIVIDUAL MAY PARTICIPATE IN ONE OR MORE FACILITIES FOLLOWING ASSESSMENT

HOSPITAL (INPATIENT)

- attend Rehabilitation Department from General Ward
- admitted to specialised psychogeriatric unit
- admitted to specialised physical rehabilitation unit

(May be moved to self-care unit prior to discharge)

DAY HOSPITAL

Transport provided to facility for treatment program

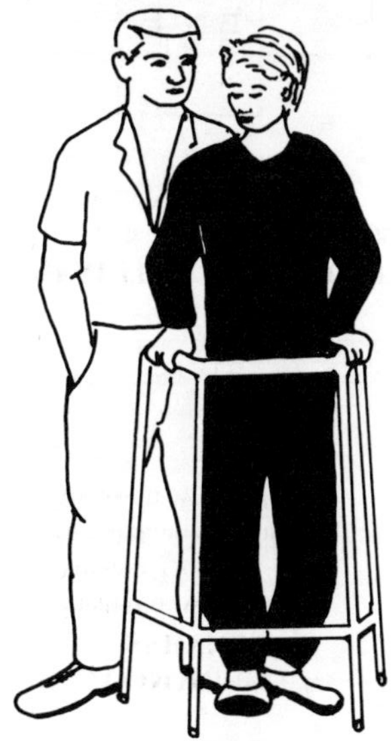

AT HOME/HOSTEL OR NURSING HOME

DAY CENTRE

Transport provided to leisure-oriented centre supervised by health professionals

COMMUNITY REHABILITATION SERVICE

Provides home-based treatment program or groups to maximise/maintain independence

GENERALIST COMMUNITY HEALTH CENTRE

Provides nursing services, advice and counselling

COMMUNITY SUPPORT SERVICES

- Home Care
- Meals-on-Wheels
- Self-help groups
- Adult leisure learning options
- Neighbourhood centres

Figure 10.5 Government and Community Services for the Elderly

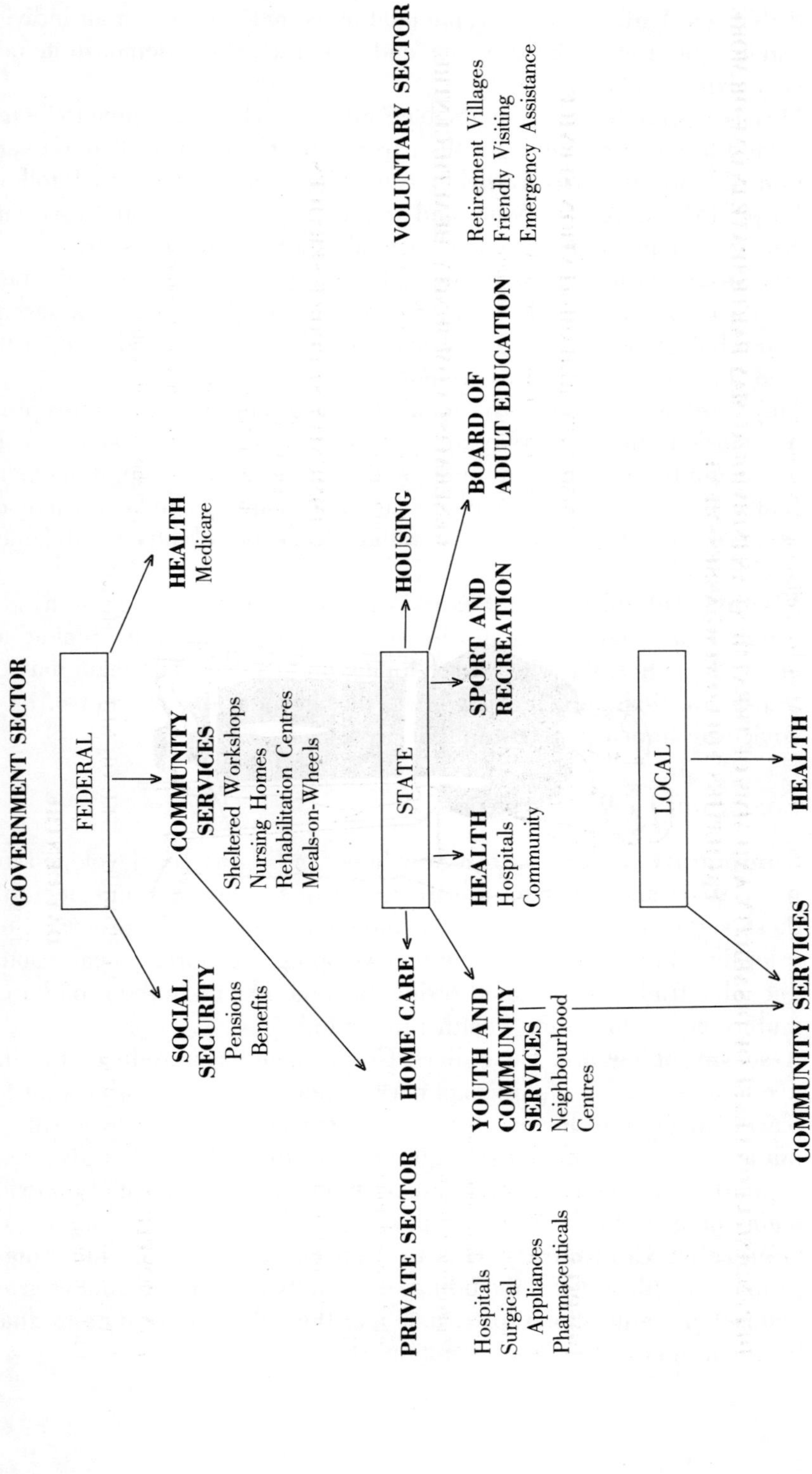

Self-Care Unit. Part of a rehabilitation complex in which an individual can live, prior to discharge home, and can practise and demonstrate necessary living skills.

Day Hospital. This service enables individuals living at home to be transported to a central point for their treatment program involving a variety of health professionals. Individuals may be referred by their GP following hospital discharge for continued treatment or for an initial assessment and treatment program when hospitalisation is unnecessary.

Psychogeriatric Rehabilitation. This is a special unit for the older person with a mental health problem. Some units provide both an assessment and rehabilitation program as well as facilities for continued care for those who do not respond to treatment.

Day Centres. Sometimes based in hospital grounds, these centres provide a leisure-oriented program supervised by a health professional. Efforts are made to maximise any independence the person may demonstrate. It also offers necessary respite for the family carers. The facility may offer programs directed towards those with a physical disability or with a mental health problem.

Visiting Rehabilitation Team. An assessment team may be available from a rehabilitation complex in the region to visit an individual at home or at a local hospital with no rehabilitation facilities. The team may offer transfer to their inpatient facilities, day hospital or day centre, or give advice on appropriate community resources.

Community health services

Community Rehabilitation Services. These services developed in the mid 1970s and focus on the treatment of the housebound person. As these services were set up under the community health program, other priorities of these services include developing appropriate local resources to enable frail aged/disabled residents to participate in the broader community and a focus on 'health promotion'.

Assessment Teams. The Federal Government has introduced this initiative to assess, on a multidisciplinary format, individuals who want to be placed in nursing homes. These assessment teams are to ensure that nursing home placement is required, and that all possible avenues for support at home have been pursued. Such teams are located on existing teams or have been set up as new services.

Generalist Community Health Centres. Provide a wide range of primary health services including community nursing, treatment groups, counselling, educational programs and the collection of data to analyse health trends in the local community.

Non-health support resources

Accommodation options

Department of Housing. Has always been quick to respond to requests for simple home modifications for an individual's needs. The Department also has a 'Special Allocations' unit and a section devoted to providing services for the disabled. In some areas the Local Authority Community Group and Housing Department have jointly established 'Group Homes' where several single people can reside, sharing a common lounge, kitchen and bathroom facilities in a home-like environment.
Hostel. This accommodation may be appropriate for some people who, due to their physical or mental health, require minimal supervision or assistance with some of the activities of daily living. Following reports such as Richmond there will be an increased demand for such services.
Nursing Home. Accommodation is available for those individuals who can no longer manage to care for themselves even with the support of available family members or community resources.
Retirement Village. Some are sponsored by religious organisations, others are operated by the private sector and offer living arrangements varying from bungalows or flats for individuals or couples to hostel areas and full nursing care sections. Individuals may need to purchase accommodation, particularly in the privately operated complexes.

Support services offered in the home

Home Care. The Home Care mandate is very broad. Some areas are able to provide a comprehensive range of services, including cleaning, shopping, ironing, supervised meal preparation and in some cases assistance with personal care or relief for carers. The demand on the service exceeds resources in some areas so they have to prioritise requests and may not be able to provide a wide range.
Meals-on-Wheels. Provide a meal delivered to the home at a minimal cost. Some districts also provide meals at a neighbourhood or community centre.
Other Services which may be available. Linen services, home handyman, gardening services, home hairdresser, home visiting craft/leisure instructors, home library service, friendly visitors.

Local community services

Neighbourhood Centres. Often run interest groups as well as providing a wide range of local information. May co-ordinate a register of local volunteers and are able to respond to occasional requests, such as accompanying someone to the doctor, dentist or optician, offering relief care or shopping services.

Adult Leisure Learning Centres. Offer a place where well and frail/disabled elderly can pursue topics of interest. May be supported by the Adult Education Board, Local Authority or Church Group. It is often essential that transport is provided to these centres.

Self-help groups

Here are some addresses of State bodies – branches of these may be found throughout Australia. This is not an exhaustive list.

- Arthritis Foundation
  12th Floor, Wynyard House,
  291 George Street,
  SYDNEY 2000.
  Tel: (02) 290 3024

- ADARDS (Alzheimer's Disease and Related Disorders Society); there is a society in every State.
  NSW contact:
  PO Box K365,
  HAYMARKET 2000
  Tel: (02) 929 4388

- Combined Pensioners Association of NSW,
  2nd Floor, 8 Kippax Street,
  SURRY HILLS 2010
  Tel: (02) 281 1811

- Multiple Sclerosis Association
  293 Mowbray Road,
  CHATSWOOD 2067
  Tel: (02) 411 4522

- ARAFMI (Association of Relatives and Friends of the Mentally Ill),
  165 Blues Point Road,
  McMAHONS POINT 2060.
  Tel: (02) 929 3192

- Better Hearing – Australia (a national organisation).
  NSW contact:
  Trades Hall, 3rd Floor,
  Cr Goulburn & Dixon Streets,
  SYDNEY 2000
  Tel: (02) 264 1305

- Epileptic Association,
  158 Pacific Highway,
  NORTH SYDNEY 2060
  Tel: (02) 920 5335

- Parkinson's Society
  NSW contact:
  Parkinson's Syndrome Society of Australia,
  PO Box 2408,
  NORTH PARRAMATTA 2151
  Tel: (02) 427 0570

- SHHH (Self-Help for Hard of Hearing People)
  PO Box 199,
  HORNSBY 2077
  Tel: (02) 48 4470
- Straight Talk and Stroke Club,
  Cleveland House,
  1 Bedford Street,
  SURRY HILLS 2010
  Tel: (02) 699 4096
- Senior Citizens Centre,
  Ring your local Council
  (See front pages of the white pages phone book).

Contact your State Council of Social Service for these services in your State.

Aids and equipment used to foster independence

A wide range of aids and equipment is available to assist individuals or families to cope following disability. Careful selection and prescription is essential.

Independent Living Centres. There are six Independent Living Centres in Australia. In addition to providing information and advice by telephone and correspondence, each centre houses a permanent exhibition of commercially available products. People can visit the Centre to try out products and make an informed choice about those which are best suited to their needs. Products are not manufactured, hired or sold at any Centre.

- ACT: Primary School, Bennelong Crescent, MACQUARIE 2614.
  Tel: (062) 51 5722.
- New South Wales: 600 Victoria Road, RYDE 2112.
  Tel: (02) 808 2233.
- Queensland: C/- Repatriation General Hospital,
  Ward 1, Newdegate Street, GREENSLOPES 4120.
  Tel: (07) 394 7471.
- South Australia: 40 Cheltenham Street, HIGHGATE 5063.
  Tel: (08) 271 1499.
- Victoria: 52 Thistlewaite Street, SOUTH MELBOURNE 3205.
  Tel: (03) 698 5290.
- Western Australia: 5 Lemnos Street, SHENTON PARK 6008.
  Tel: (09) 382 2011.

Program of Aids for Disabled People (PADP). In 1981 a previous system administered through YACS (Youth and Community Services) was expanded and reorganised and is now available via the Health Department through local hospitals. It provides aids and equipment for long-term use in the home. The system is not strictly means-tested, but details are requested about a household's financial circumstances and each hospital sets its own criteria. This system is not available for people residing in a nursing home.

Equipment Leading Pools (ELP). Most rehabilitation facilities can organise the initial short-term loan of equipment from area ELPs, such as mobility aids, frames or wheelchairs and personal care items such as bath aids. Contact your Health Department Regional Office, local hospital or community health centre for exact details.

Technical Aid to the Disabled (TAD). Comprises administrative staff and a group of volunteers with engineering and technical skills. In the absence of a suitable commercially available aid, the volunteers will design, construct, adapt, install and maintain aids for people who are disabled. TAD operates in every State and Territory, with the exception of Western Australia.

- New South Wales: PO Box 108, RYDE 2112.
  Tel: (02) 808 2022.
- ACT: RM901 Burra Road, LITTLE BURRA 2620.
  Tel: (062) 36 3129.
- Victoria: PO Box 88, SOUTH MELBOURNE 3205.
  Tel: (03) 698 5290.
- Queensland: PO Box 127, SPRING HILL 4000.
  Tel: (07) 229 2822 Ext 296.
- Northern Territory: 21 Savannah Drive, LEANDER 5793.
  Tel: (089) 27 1166.
- Tasmania: PO Box 155, BELLERIVE 7018.
  Tel: (002) 28 8319.

Conclusion

This chapter demonstrates the important role played by the nurse in the historical development of rehabilitation. It has also focused on the present contribution of the nurse in the team approach. The team concept and the appropriate use of resources relate closely to the success of the rehabilitation process. Success also depends on a knowledge of the individual's experience of this process. These comments highlight the needs of elderly consumers and the potential challenges for workers in this field.

Questions

1. What is the philosophy behind current rehabilitation practice?
2. What is the unique contribution of the nurse in the rehabilitation process?
3. How does the nurse's role interact with others in the approach?
4. Compare the differences between interdisciplinary and multidisciplinary approaches and evaluate their worth in terms of individual/client care.
5. Describe the rehabilitation process from the personal and bureaucratic perspectives.
6. Describe the issues facing the older person in their interactions with workers.
7. What is the challenge of working with the elderly?

References

1. Websters New Collegiate Dictionary. Springfield: G and C Merriam Co, 1973.
2. Nightingale F. Notes on nursing. What it is, and what it is not. New York: Dover Publications, Inc, 1969.
3. Henderson V. Basic principles of nursing care. Switzerland: International Council of Nurses, 1977.
4. Wilson HS, Kneisl CR. Psychiatry nursing. Menlo Park, California: Addison-Wesley, 1983.
5. McGilloway FA. Dependency and vulnerability in the nurse/patient relationship. Journal of Advanced Nursing 1976; 1: 3.
6. Avorn J, Langer F. Induced disability in nursing home patients. Journal of American Geriatric Society 1983: 30.
7. Yarmesh M, Sheafor M. The decision to restrain. Geriatric Nursing 1984.
8. Lancely A. Use of controlling language in rehabilitation. Journal of Advanced Nursing 1985:11.
9. Willis E. Sister Elizabeth Kenny and the evolution of the occupational division of labour in health care. Australian and New Zealand Journal of Sociology 1979; 15(3).
10. Adcock W et al. With courage and devotion: a history of midwifery in NSW. Melbourne: Royal Australian Nursing Federation, 1984.
11. Melvin JL. Interdisciplinary and multidisciplinary activities and ACRM. Archives of Physical and Medical Rehabilitation 1980: 61.
12. Rothberg JS. The rehabilitation team: future directions. Archives of Physical and Medical Rehabilitation 1981: 62.

13. Henderson V. Prescribing the essence of nursing in a technological age. Journal of Advanced Nursing 1980; 5(3).

Further reading

Arndt K, Teterycz P, Valentin L. Interdisciplinary rehabilitation modules. Supervisory Nurse 1978 9(2).

Bandura A. Principles of behaviour modification. New York: Holt, Rhinehart and Winston, 1969.

Bandura A. Social learning theory. New York: Holt, Rhinehart and Winston, 1977.

Brodsky I. Sydney's nurse crusaders. Sydney: Old Sydney Free Press, 1968.

Correll D. The multidisciplinary approach to rehabilitation. Australian Family Physician 1981: 10.

Eisenberg MG, Griggens C, Duval RJ. Disabled people as second-class citizens. New York: Springer Publishing Co, 1982.

Grief E, Matarazzo RG. Behavioural approaches to rehabilitation. New York: Springer Publishing Co, 1982.

Hall I. One hundred years of army nursing. London: Cassell and Co, 1953.

Hetzel BS. Health and Australian society. Melbourne: Penguin Books Australia Ltd, 1977.

Jackson O, ed. Physical therapy of the geriatric patient. Edinburgh: Churchill Livingstone, 1983.

Leventhal N. Interdisciplinary teamwork: a crucial dimension in rehabilitation therapy. American Archives of Rehabilitation Therapy 1975 23(2).

McQueen H. Social sketches of Australia: 1888-1975. Sydney: Penguin Books Australia, 1978.

Maddison D, Day P, Leabeater B. Psychiatric nursing. London: Churchill Livingstone, 1967.

Russell C. Studies in society. The ageing experience. Australia: George Allen and Unwin, 1981.

Sainsbury MJ. Key to psychiatry. Sydney: ANZ Book Co, 1976.

Test MA, Stein LI. A community approach to the chronically disabled patient. Social Policy 1977 8(1).

Vash CL. The psychology of disability. New York: Springer Publishing Co, 1981.

Chapter 11

Activities for the Aged in Supervised Accommodation, Hospitals or Activity Centres

Objectives

To enable the reader to:

1. identify physiological, psychological and sociological problems of the aged and discuss these in relation to activities;
2. identify and discuss issues that will affect the selection and organisation of activities for the aged;
3. identify and discuss a range of activities suitable for the aged within supervised care accommodation and activity centres;
4. identify and discuss some of the specific activity needs of the aged presenting with confusion and memory loss;
5. discuss the roles of a nurse in relation to activity programs for the aged when:
   (a) in a support role;
   (b) as the activity leader.

There is no such ethnic or social group as 'the aged', only individuals from all groups, with vast differences and personalities, who have grown old. Thus, their needs for activity will vary widely. People should not be categorised by chronological age, but by functional age.

While theoretically no one is disabled by age itself, inevitably the continuous physical and psychological processes associated with ageing take their toll. There are many negative factors that need to be considered as these have important implications for one's approach to the provision of activities for the aged.

Negative aspects of age

An aged person may have:

- reduced self-esteem, loss of self-identity and dignity. This is particularly noticeable in institutions where there may be a lack of privacy, individuality, or freedom of movement;
- reduced social skills;
- reduced attention span, short-term memory loss;
- slower reaction times, so the aged become more cautious because of a fear of accidents;
- confusion and disorientation – precipitated by changes in accommodation, modes of living, unfamiliar routines, and lack of family and social supports;
- decreased mobility, a slow gait, unstable balance, awkward walking aids, painful feet;
- impaired manual dexterity due to limited joint ranges, inco-ordination and muscle weakness;
- reduced tolerances of change, discomfort and fatigue due to the body's diminished ability to adapt – particularly to temperature extremes;
- diminished perception due to sensory loss:
  - hearing loss accounts for lost ability to communicate effectively, and wearing hearing aids may mean an intolerance of background noise;
  - visual impairment may mean the loss of enjoyable interests such as reading, and an intolerance of glare. Good illumination will be required;
  - taste impairments increase the loss of interest in food;
- increased introspection, lessened consideration of others;
- structure hunger – meaning a need for routine, familiar surroundings, timetables and organisation of their time;
- reduced motivation for activity – usually means most of their other needs have already been met in their earlier life, e.g. family, financial security;

- a tendency to withdraw from their usual activities as part of a denial of the increasing deterioration of their abilities;
- a fear of failure or ridicule, particularly in simple activities;
- a fear that exertion will precipitate a medical disaster or pain;
- financial insecurity and feelings of being an economic burden;
- feelings of being useless and unproductive;
- increased need for spiritual support.[1-3]

Issues affecting the aged

The ageing person has developed attitudes and opinions that have been formed and cemented over many years of vast and varied experiences. Some of these have been very unpleasant such as wars, and the Depression. These attitudes and sometimes prejudices should be acknowledged and the right to hold these views respected.

There exists a gap of at least two generations between most nurses and the ageing person they care for. With this gap tremendous alterations in the familiar Australian culture have occurred, due to advances in technology and the contribution of our migrants. It is always important for the younger carer to remember that a concept they take for granted may be almost alien to an aged person.

Western culture has placed an increasing emphasis on the value of productivity, activity and consumption.[1,3] For the majority of aged people their work has been the greatest influence in structuring their use of time. Their remaining hours were spent largely in sleeping, eating and preparation for the next day. Free time is a relatively new concept for the aged.

This work ethos also influenced the use of leisure time. Our culture has tended to value productive leisure as more praiseworthy than passive recreational pursuits. For example, charitable works, hobbies and gardening are held in more esteem than sitting in a park, chatting to a friend, or listening to a record. Aged people have been condemned to live in a perpetual state of leisure and have no defined effective or satisfactory role in our society.[4]

Some factors which prevent the ageing person from feeling productive and a contributing member of society are enforced retirement at lower ages due to technological advances, reduced financial income, shorter work hours, smaller nuclear families, a tendency for the aged to live separately from their families, and increased life expectancies.

Appropriate activities can help the aged person feel that life is still worth living. They can provide goals, praise for achievements, opportunities to use remaining skills, a sense of well-being, social contacts and proof that their past experiences are still valuable to them.

Scheduled group and individual activities should:

- be designed to make life more meaningful;
- stimulate and support a desire to use the aged person's physical and mental capabilities to their fullest extent;
- maintain their highest attainable social, physical and emotional function;
- provide a sense of usefulness and self-respect;
- be suited to the aged person's individual needs.[4(p 452)]

Assessment for activity

Activity for activity's sake is no longer acceptable. Each patient should be interviewed, goals established with that patient and activities planned which contribute to these goals.

When involving the aged in any activity the unique qualities of each person must be recognised and respected. First, get to know them, discover their interests, hobbies, jobs, where they lived, and their social background so that they can be more readily involved in something that will be of interest to them. By talking to the staff and family, one can discover the aged person's abilities and disabilities, whether they are gregarious or a loner, and how they cope with their activities of daily living.

The time spent in assessing and knowing the person behind the disability is also invaluable in building trust in relationships between the aged person and the activity leader.[2] It is also essential to assess fully the physical environment, including routines and attitudes of the other staff and helpers, before beginning an activity.

Implementation of an activity program

When introducing an activity program or even one new activity, it is important that all concerned understand fully what is involved. The institution's management must be conversant with the aims of the program and know it is not usually a self-financing project. An activity leader is not there primarily to raise funds but to reactivate the aged group in the facility.

Explanation is needed as to how the frail aged will benefit (e.g. by their improved quality of life), how nursing can ultimately be made easier and more interesting, and how staff can assist. This can prevent the frustration of interruptions in an activity with the ensuing loss of group cohesion that often occurs.

Support staff also need explanations as to why there may be a necessity for moving furniture, changes to routines, increased untidiness and interruption to usual cleaning programs. These explanations should ideally come from the matron (or supervisor) so naturally she should be fully informed about the activity program.

The types and range of activities will depend on:

- the type of facility, e.g. hostel, day centre, club, nursing home;
- the needs of that aged group in the facility;
- the number and skills of the activity leaders;
- the amount of support from other staff;
- the resources available within the facility and the local community.

Aims of an activity program

An activity program for the aged should:

- offer a range of activities to utilise the widely differing skills and personalities of the aged and encourage them to participate;
- provide opportunities to maintain and increase their level of independence and do as much as possible despite the limitations of their disabilities;
- provide new acquaintances to help fill the gaps left by bereavement and separation from their children and peers;
- help the older person to keep fit, thus helping to maintain the health process. It may also be a useful intervention strategy where breakdown in health has occurred;
- structure the day, fill in the long idle hours purposefully, thus maintaining good morale and controlling introspection;
- revive old skills, thus reinforcing the notion that existing abilities are valuable. The aged have assets that are often forgotten, mostly underplayed, and always underutilised;
- provide opportunities to learn new skills to replace those that are no longer applicable or physically possible;
- supply an outlet for the basic need to help others, particularly for those who have always been carers themselves, thus fulfilling the need to be useful;

- improve and maintain self-identity and a high self-esteem. It is the recognition of personal achievements that establishes status in the eyes of ourselves, our peers, and juniors.
- provide, through exercise, the physiological benefits of improved respiratory and circulatory activity, elimination, appetite, sleep patterns and maintenance of joint ranges and muscle strengths at optimum levels;
- provide an immediate sense of involvement and enjoyable anticipation of future events.[3]

Types of activities

Activities can be either passive or active, stimulating or relaxing, structured or unstructured, productive or creative, require social interaction or be solitary, but are more usually a combination of these.

There are nine basic types of activities.[3] These are:

- Physical – exercises, bowls
- Mental – discussion, table games
- Individual – sewing, jigsaws, letter writing
- Small group – cards, committees, chatting to others
- Social – parties, singalongs
- Service to others – fund-raising, helping
- Cultural – craft, music
- Spiritual – church, prayer, reading
- Daily living activities – dressing, eating.

Group activities

Appropriate and effective group participation should be encouraged. This is because groups are a more economical use of an activity leader's time and also an integral part of our society. Several needs can usually be met at once in a group situation, e.g. social interaction and physical exercise can be happily incorporated in party games.

Start with a small group of six, then increase to twelve; an optimum group size at any one time in a program will be between fourteen and twenty-two.[1(p 8)] More than twenty-two tends to require a major effort to organise satisfactorily if there is only one person and creates a feeling of impersonality.

The group process itself can be therapeutic as it offers an opportunity for peer involvement, social interaction, an identity, and an opportunity to share problems. Some people find participating as a member of a group less threatening than as an individual. As the elderly may have already experienced upheavals from the disintegration of their familiar social supports, joining a group can fulfil a need for belonging.

Organisation

These are the important points to consider when organising a program of activities for the aged.

- Start slowly with passive activities such as films, music and entertainment which will encourage participation without having to prove oneself.
- Be content with only a few participants. Remember the fringe dwellers will be stimulated despite initially not actively participating.
- Never pressure anyone into taking part and continue to maintain a friendly rapport, whether they participate or not. Continuous, gentle persuasion can often work wonders.
- Some people always like to be invited to join in.
- Start with 'normal' types of activities that the group may have enjoyed before coming to the institution, e.g. picnics, cards, afternoon teas.
- Alternate unstructured activities like morning tea with 'active' things such as exercise groups.
- Remember it is not necessary to have everyone constantly occupied or busy as the attention span of the aged is often shortened.
- Be flexible and prepared to alter the program, e.g. to accommodate changes of mood, weather, resources. It is often easier for the leader to adapt than the aged person.
- Never do anything for them that they can do themselves, including making decisions. Remember to offer a choice in activities.
- Set realistic achievable goals.
- Speak clearly, give clear instructions and allow time for their response. If required, repeat the instruction. When possible, use an example of the process at each stage and, importantly, the finished project. Remember to be a good listener.
- Exercise patience, tact, tolerance, and respect their confidences.
- Always emphasise their abilities, not disabilities. Be positive, show enthusiasm, and remember to give praise and encouragement. Motivation comes from within, and the best stimulation comes from recognition of achievement.

- Avoid unnecessary distractions, particularly those due to noise or physical discomfort.
- Use aids to help orientate the person as part of the normal program, and in subtle ways include it in conversation.
- Try to spend time equally with each individual.
- Create an atmosphere of acceptance, warmth and cheerfulness.
- Provide structure by a planned routine of activities but include something new at least each week. However, completely abandon structure for special occasions like films, guest speakers, holidays and celebrations.
- The elderly in general do not enjoy activities that are particularly messy, dirty or very noisy.
- Allow for movement by changing activities every 30 minutes or so (40 minutes maximum). Most of the aged become stiff and restless if they must remain in one spot for long periods of time. Very energetic or demanding activities should be of short duration (5 minutes).
- Be aware of specific disabilities and adapt the activity or equipment as required. If changing rules of well known games, call them by different names to lessen confusion.
- Always respect group members' dignity and individuality by being understanding and non-judgmental and try to be sensitive to their unmet needs or unexpressed fears.[2]

Timing and structure

Social pressures have moulded most of us to accept the community's timetable for meals, work, chores and recreation at set intervals. Fear of solitude and idleness encourages people to build a time structure even into their leisure persuits. Consequently, most people learn to interrupt one activity in favour of another. Time itself can then become more important than the activity, thus making leisure time hard to occupy with anything other than short bursts of interest. Years of living to timetables have left the aged particularly with a need for structured use of time.

Thus, many people regard guided activity as being more acceptable than finding ways to occupy themselves. To be satisfied with the activity program, the aged person must recognise a structure that is familiar to them, and also see it as worthwhile. Therefore, in institutional settings, it is important to program the day with activities that at times reflect the person's usual way of life.[1,3]

Environmental resources

A balanced program will be interesting, stimulating and motivating. It will involve as many amenities and community resources as possible, and also other staff, health professionals, the members themselves and their families. Volunteers, if willing to accept direction, can be a valuable asset to any program.

The area where the activities take place does not need to be grand. The basic requirements are adequate heating in winter, ventilation in summer, and freedom from draughts.[1] Preferably, there should be no steps, and the floor surface should be non-slippery. Good lighting without glare and accessible toilets are essential.

Stable chairs with arms, and tables of the correct height that can be moved easily for more vigorous activities, are required for most centres. Ideally, there should be a storage area, and an area or kitchen for food preparation. One should be able to isolate or confine noisy or messy activities easily. Display boards, a clock, mirrors and a day/date calendar are advisable.

Support role of the nurse

In the majority of cases, the nurse will not be designated the activity program leader, but she still has a vital role to support the leader both directly and indirectly. In many institutions the diversional therapist works only part-time and thus it is even more important for the nurse to consolidate the activity program.

Nurses should not confuse their role as a care giver with that required by an activity leader. By giving priority to their nursing role during an activity group, nurses may inadvertently reinforce the patient's role of being sick and dependent as more important than the healthier role of an active group participant. Administering medication and medical treatment during groups are examples of this. The intrinsic involvement with the intimate areas of hygiene, toileting and listening to personal problems is acknowledged by society as being within the professional role of a nurse. It is important to remember that such an involvement in the private concerns of a person is at variance with the normal levels of social propriety, other than those of the family or spouse.

The nurse should be aware of the patient's sensitivity to such matters and the dilemma of the duality of roles when acting as both a nurse and the activity leader. A nurse, other than the activity leader, should deal with the toileting needs of the patient in order to maintain the patient's dignity and enable a more normal social relationship in activity groups.

When in a support role, the nurse should try to:

- inform the activity leader of any emotional and medical occurrences that may alter the performance of the group members, e.g. alterations to medication such as the increasing of diuretics may affect their ability to go on an outing; or special dietary needs such as those for diabetics; or special medical problems such as limited exercise tolerances, confusion, and a tendency to wander;
- inform the activity leader of the known medical problems which may interfere with the member's participation, thus enabling activities to be modified to eliminate unnecessary failure and frustration by the participant;
- inform the leader of each group participant's level of independence, particularly, for example, with meals and toileting, which may directly influence their ability to participate in outings;
- help in physically collecting the participants of the group;
- ensure each member is ready to participate by wearing glasses, hearing aids, and clothing appropriate to the activity;
- be generous with praise and recognise the participant's achievements regardless of how limited they may seem;
- provide encouragement before and during the group for those members who are hesitant;
- encourage and support those members who are limited by physical disabilities such as arthritis, poor vision or memory loss, in the various games and activities;
- consolidate the group's ideas by maintaining interest after the activity is over by, for example, continuing group discussion themes, or framing an art class project, or helping with a craft;
- provide encouragement for the whole activity program and respect the work being done by the diversional therapist;
- harmonise the aims of the activity program with those of the institution;
- develop a close relationship with the diversional therapist/activity leader by:
  - discussing together the aims of the groups;
  - providing an interchange of ideas between the different disciplines;
  - joint program planning;
  - analysing the outcomes of the groups;
- be aware of the contribution the diversional therapist can make in the reporting of the participant's progress. A reported change in

behaviour, for example, may assist the early detection of an infection. Participation in an activity program can give valuable insight into the capabilities of the person behind their presenting patient role;

- maintain confidentiality, as group members often relate pertinent information during the relaxed atmosphere of an informal gathering.

Activities of daily living

It is no kindness to 'over-nurse' a person, as feelings of uselessness and loss of self-respect increase as a person becomes more dependent. Even the simple activity of walking helps to maintain proper elimination, balance, and the senses, and to improve circulation and respiration.[5] When exercise is inadequate, muscles atrophy and joints stiffen. So it is vital to stimulate the aged and keep whatever physical capabilities they still have, and to maintain optimum independence in the activities of daily living, such as feeding, grooming, bathing, toileting and handling money.

Each patient should be assessed and realistic goals set, and all staff must maintain a consistent approach if the person is to reach these. We often do not expect enough of the aged because of their disabilities. Pressures such as lack of staff and time commitments overrule their needs, and the time required to enable self-help. This may involve risks and increased work for the nurse, e.g. spills from self-feeding.

One of the greatest restorers of self-esteem for the handicapped is that of regaining their independence, including maintenance of privacy in their personal hygiene and toileting. Advice about incontinence aids and suitable clothing can be one simple measure to ensure the aged continue to attend activities.

Remember that, due to disabilities, new methods may have to be taught for the simplest activities that would previously have been done automatically. It is usually necessary to demonstrate the technique one step at a time. This is particularly the case when verbal communication has been affected, as in a stroke or with a confused person. The aged person must experience at least partial success if they are to persist.

Clothing and grooming are an important reinforcer of identity and self-esteem. The aged should be complimented on their appearance and encouraged to take pride in it again. Visits to the hairdresser, a new garment to wear, manicuring their nails, light application of makeup, or even simply rubbing in hand cream will certainly encourage an aged woman to maintain her appearance.

If the aged are to be encouraged to remain independent the physical environment should not be inhibiting. Some of the things that may mean the difference between dependency and self-help are rails at correct heights, arms on chairs that are not too low, lever handles on taps and doors, doors that are not too heavy to open, and special eating utensils or crockery. An occupational therapist will be able to provide advice about suitable aids or adaptations for activities of daily living and for most recreational activities.

Productive activities

Craft

Craft work is not universally popular. In fact, many of the aged have never been interested in craft work or manual skills. 'Making things' is often rated quite low by the aged when discussing their interests.[3] Despite this, most institutions overemphasise this aspect of a program. This is probably due to the tangible evidence that finished goods provide, and their potential for revenue making. Craft activities should always be optional but be part of a program available for those who want them.

It is often found that the aged express no need to produce items for themselves but enjoy doing so for others (e.g. their family, fund-raising, charitable groups). In many craft groups, people participate as much for the company and interaction itself. Other aged people actively avoid craft as it may frustrate them by highlighting their inability to continue with previous skills which may have been of a very high level. It is important to stress to the aged person that in any craft, perfection, quality and quantity are secondary to simply being absorbed in doing and creating something with one's own hands. To lose self-consciousness for a time through absorption in manual, creative activity can be an immensely refreshing and relaxing phenomenon.[1]

However, free expression, experimentation and other abstract concepts in crafts are not familiar to the aged. They prefer concrete concepts and do not enjoy creativity as an end in itself. Thus, any finished craft product should be useful and be of a reasonable standard of workmanship. It should not appear childish or use materials and equipment similar to those used by their grandchildren.

All activities should be well prepared and the instructor should have a good understanding of the processes involved. Most importantly, as much as possible of the work should be done by the aged person with minimal intervention from the instructor.

Selected crafts for the aged should always be:

- structured;
- repetitive of technique;
- made of easily obtainable materials at an affordable price;

- obviously useful in the eyes of the elderly;
- colourful and larger than normal, as these are easier to manipulate than very small items;
- not too large or heavy for easy handling;
- fairly clean and non-sticky;
- within the person's capacity;
- attractive and of a reasonable standard of workmanship;
- require minimal staff preparation or finishing time;
- not reliant on fine steady movements, e.g. jewellery;
- not reliant on speed (sewing machines are often too fast);
- interesting, enjoyable, and foster a sense of achievement.[3(p 29)]

Successful craft items are generally simple, quick to complete, and require minimum preparation and finishing by the instructor, who is there to guide, not to manufacture.

Gardening

This is a popular interest of the aged. Ideally, the heavy work of digging and the group work of planting should be minimal. Long-handled tools, special kneeling chairs and commercially available raised garden beds can help overcome some of the problems.

Alternatively, the aged could be encouraged to plant into tubs and pots, strike cuttings, start seedlings for the hospital garden, start window boxes of herbs, grow bean sprouts, and plants in water and terrariums. Flower arranging and pressing dry flowers are two popular associated gardening activities.

Workshop

Simple workshop activities and repairs are also enjoyed by the elderly. These can range from simple sanding of wooden toys and aids to upholstery and repairing hospital furniture. A separate area should be designated for these activities because of the risk of paint fumes, dust and noise. All activities should be supervised as there is always the potential for accidents with confused patients who may use tools inappropriately.

Cooking

Simple recipes, particularly those requiring no cooking, are usually successful. The aged should be encouraged to help cater for special events, or even just provide a cake or sandwiches for an informal gathering of friends. A cooking workshop, e.g. making marmalade or recipe swapping, is also enjoyable.

Work-oriented activities

Industrial therapy, or work-related activity, is a controversial issue. There is a dilemma between the accusation of exploitation and the possible benefits to those aged who prefer useful work rather than games and craft. There are many routine clerical activities that could be used, such as folding, stapling and stamping.[3] It is important that the aged person is not pressured to meet deadlines and that disproportionate amounts of staff time are not used in preparation and checking.

Creative activities

Art

With encouragement, many aged people can enjoy art classes, but the subject matter should always be clearly defined. Water-soluble, non-toxic paints are an ideal medium, and collages can sometimes be a way of encouraging group participation. Discussion can arise during the art class or can occur at the end of the session.

Mental stimulation

It is now easier to present quizzes because of the popularity of current television panel games, and very physically disabled members can be encouraged to participate competitively in mental activities. Ideally, groups should be kept small.

A few suggestions are crosswords, debates, word games, general knowledge and problem solving. These can be organised on an individual or team basis.

Discussion groups

These are a good medium for encouraging interaction, and building identity and self-esteem. Unless hampered by a disability, most of the aged have communication skills which are highly developed. Encouraging them to draw on past experiences and to relate these to current affairs can help orientate the confused person. The group could also make a valuable resource folder, say for a historical group.

Smedley[6] proposes that, when organising a discussion group, one should consider the following points:

- make the topic clear;
- listen to all contributions, assist anyone not expressing himself clearly;
- be sincere;
- be flexible in your point of view, don't argue;
- don't tell anyone they are wrong, or ridicule them;
- don't monopolise, talk too loudly or too long;
- don't be too serious;
- set time limits.

Some suggestions for topics are current affairs, work, favourite hobbies, holidays.

Table games

Card games, draughts, dominoes, bingo and scrabble are the most popular table games. Many of the aged find closer companionship provided by these smaller groups. However, it is important to remember that onlookers tend to feel left out. It is also important that rules be established at the beginning, as many aged are unable or unwilling to alter the playing rules they have fostered all their lives.

Passive activity

Initially, many members prefer to participate in passive activities only, as these are less threatening. It is important that these do not last too long. Slides and travel films, concerts and music groups are very popular. Being read to can be very therapeutic as it is relaxing and encourages active listening (10 to 15 minutes recommended time).

Exercise

Most aged people enjoy and need little persuasion to join exercise groups. Little preparation or financial outlay is required by the instructor. However, she does need to convey a light-hearted but confident approach, preferably without resorting to written notes.[3]

Most of the exercises should be done while seated, and there should be enough room to stretch without touching others. The exercise session should last 20 minutes, preferably with a break midway. Participants should be watched for signs of distress. It is rare for the elderly to overextend themselves, as most are aware of their limitations. A good guide is whether the elderly can maintain normal conversation during the exercise session.

Participation should always be optional. The leader should be ready to explain the benefits of each of the exercises. Variety can be obtained by adding new exercises, and by using props such as music, balls, scarves, balloons and beanbags.

The exercise group is a good opportunity to incorporate recreational games such as quoits, beanbags toss or balloon volley ball. Exercise groups should take place before main meals, and include breathing and relaxation exercises. Relaxation is very important for the elderly, as it can decrease levels of pain, anxiety and insomnia. Walking is a particularly good exercise. At every opportunity, when good weather prevails, the elderly should take short walks outside the buildings.

Physical games

Points to consider when using physical games with the aged:

- Wear clothing that does not hinder, e.g. correct shoes for bowls.
- Use those popular games that are familiar and recognised by the community, such as bowls, pool, croquet, skittles, darts, quoits.
- Use games that are adult in type and presentation. Reserve the more simple, fun games for party days where they will be enjoyed and seen as socially acceptable.
- Wherever possible, use standard rules and equipment. If changing these, call the game by another name.
- Explain all rules before beginning and maintain strict fairness when scoring, or else don't score.
- Games can channel competitiveness, give a feeling of camaraderie and belonging if a team spirit emerges.
- Non-participants may still enjoy being spectators, or assist as scorers.[3]

Music

Music is enjoyed by nearly everyone as it brings pleasure to even the severely mentally impaired. Live music is particularly appreciated. Music has the ability to relax, and evoke past memories of happiness and sorrow. Singalongs of hymns and old songs lead to a feeling of good cheer and can alleviate depression and loneliness. Music can even distract from chronic pain.

Participation can be in many forms, such as accompanying with percussion instruments, waving scarves, moving in time, tapping hands or feet, or even simple reflective listening.

However, despite all the advantages of music, there are some people who have a sensitivity to noise and will become agitated. Pianolas are often not enjoyed as they are too loud. All participants should be asked if they object to music playing, and asked for their musical preferences.

Special events

Special occasions such as celebrations, parties, demonstrations and barbecues can provide opportunities to:

- use the variety of catering skills of the aged;
- provide a variety of foods which can be enjoyed;
- use social skills and meet different people;
- have pleasure and fun with new games and activities;
- raise funds;
- involve larger groups, particularly for concerts;
- get dressed up;
- vary the program and involve many members usefully in the planning, preparing decorations, and setting up stages;
- provide something to look forward to.

Individual activities

The aged can be encouraged to continue craft activities after hours once they are familiar with the techniques. Other individual pursuits could include reading, writing to friends, writing to their family, history, exercise, walking, gardening, telephoning friends and shopping for someone more disabled.

Others prefer an activity involving responsibility such as caring for plants, arranging the flowers, keeping club records or a diary for the activity centre.

Outings

Consider these points when arranging an outing.

- Even many of the active aged have lost confidence and severely limit their visits out into the community.
- Group outings involve considerable advance planning and care.
- Toilets must be accessible.

- The presence of steps and a suitable ground surface are important, e.g. it is difficult to walk on grass with sticks.
- The distance involved from the venue to the transport drop-off point and provision for parking the vehicle.
- The availability of seats within an exhibition being visited.
- Are the costs affordable?
- Take first aid kit and be aware of special medical requirements.
- Extra staff and helpers are usually required.
- Suitable transport for staff and helpers and mobility aids.
- Arrangements and preparation for meals in advance.
- Inform the group so that they are correctly dressed.
- Duration of activity and opening times of the venue need to be checked.

Dementia and related problems

An activities program for people with dementia is quite different from one for the mentally alert frail aged. People with dementia present as confused and with severe memory loss. They need a warm, friendly atmosphere within a secure environment, and very simple, non-threatening familiar activities that are within their capabilities. The emphasis is on maintaining their remaining physical skills, and the rediscovery of memories to help them maintain their sense of personal identity.

Points to consider when planning activities with the confused aged with memory loss are:

- use orientation aids and techniques;
- activities should be familiar, self-explanatory, one step at a time, and be completed in a short time;
- maintain routines, as the confused are unable to adapt easily to changes;
- avoid clutter;
- the emphasis is on normal activities of daily life, with simple, routine, domestic tasks;
- utilise and reinforce existing skills rather than try to teach new skills;
- music, physical recreation and exercise groups have proved highly successful with this group;
- elements of orientation, remotivation and reminiscence programs can be incorporated to encourage the demented person to relate and redevelop feelings of self-identity.

Therapeutic activities

Reality orientation – since dementia is associat
and disorientation, a reality orientation approach s
patients. Reality orientation is based on the assumpt
information, i.e. patient's name, place, time of day, day o
name of next meal and special events, can reinforce learning and ameliorate disorientation and confusion.

RO techniques should be used within the day centre and given naturally and consistently in the course of conversation by all staff. The four sign-posts used to help prevent people getting lost in their confusion are:

- **who** – patient is always addressed by their preferred name.
- **where** – the place the activity will occur.
- **what** – what is going to happen next.
- **when** – at what time this will happen.

E.g. Mrs Smith **(who)**, would you like to come to the dining room **(where)** for lunch **(what)**, now? **(when)**[7]

Often it is most important, when you are greeting patients on arrival, for the driver to say to them: "Here is Mrs Atkinson." You may then say: "Good morning, Mrs Smith, you're looking nice today. Please come inside the day centre for a cup of tea." A similar procedure would occur at the end of the day, when they would be told of the next visit.

It is more usual in a day centre to use the RO techniques for the whole group at once, e.g. "At 11 o'clock when you have all finished this game, we will move into the next room for the morning exercise group with Mrs Atkinson."

The equipment needed for reality orientation includes:

- large clock;
- clear day/date/year calendar, name of organisation;
- simple daily program, arrival and departure times;
- areas obviously labelled, e.g. toilet;
- map of locality on wall.

All staff, volunteers and patients should wear name tags.

Attitude therapy is another approach. This is a consistent rehabilitation team approach which is helpful in reinforcing desirable behaviour and eliminating undesirable behaviour.

Life review (or reminiscing groups) is a process of actively encouraging recall of the past to help other people evaluate the meaning of their lives.[8]

miniscence therapy:

- attempts to cater for the psychological needs of the elderly;
- creates a climate where members can rediscover a sense of worth and identity;
- acknowledges the individual as unique and with valuable past experiences.

The family's involvement in producing a 'This is your Life' sheet and book are invaluable, both for staff and patient.[9] In stimulating reminiscence, audio-visual aids and documentary records of war days could be starting points. Local historical societies, visits to antique stores or old work places could also provoke memories.

It is difficult to organise specific groups within an integrated day centre – often these techniques are incorporated informally in group discussions.

Remotivation is a technique that encourages moderately confused older individuals to become more interested in their surroundings and strengthens their ability to communicate and socialise with others. It capitalises on the patient's long memory store (their prime time of life being 1920-1945) and aims to bring them up to date with comparison of then and now. All the senses are stimulated and a wealth of memory aids are utilised, e.g. old photos, antiques, books, films. A remotivation group is a formal procedure consisting of five steps and lasting 50 minutes.

Organisation of a remotivation group involves:

- five minutes to develop a climate of acceptance;
- fifteen minutes to build a bridge to reality, often in the form of a poem, famous quotation, or newspaper item;
- fifteen minutes in developing the topic to be covered by the group, called 'Sharing the World we Live In'. An effective method of fostering interest is to use related props, e.g. photos, samples.
- fifteen minutes to design an appreciation of the work of the world, to prompt the patient into thinking about work in relation to himself;
- five minutes spent in the climate of appreciation to summarise and arrange the next meeting.

Conclusion

The substance of this chapter applies only to a minority (25 per cent) of the ageing population, of whom only 5 per cent are currently in long-care institutions. The vast majority of the aged (at least 75 per cent) are fully independent and living in the community.

It is now widely recognised that maintaining or developing substantial levels of physical, mental and social activity contributes to successful ageing. To this end, the independent aged are involved in a variety of organisations such as senior citizens, sports clubs, hobby classes, church groups, fund-raising charitable groups and interest groups. They engage in individual pursuits, and contribute to the growing success of various healthy lifestyle programs for the older person.

Questions

1. What negative factors may affect the approach to and provision of activities for the aged?
2. Describe the effect of Western culture on the older person's use of time.
3. Hopkins (1978) identifies five goals for scheduled group and individual activities. What are they?
4. Discuss the place of assessment in planning an activity program.
5. Identify the factors which determine the types and range of activities that might be carried out with older patients.
6. List six aims of an activity program for the aged.
7. What are the nine basic types of activities which may be used in programs for older people?
8. List six important points to consider when organising an activity program.
9. Why is the structuring of time so important in activity programs?
10. Explore the nurse's role in activities programs.
11. In what ways does an activities program for the older person with dementia differ from that for other older people?

References

1. McHarg M. Activity clubs for frail and handicapped persons. Sydney: Hornsby and Ku-ring-gai Area Health Centre, 1980.
2. Blackett L. Involving the aged – craft and activities for the disabled. Paper presented at the Australian Association of Geriatric Nursing Activity Conference, Sydney, 1980.
3. Cornish PM. Activities for the frail aged. Sydney, 1975.
4. Hopkins HL, Smith HD. Willard and Spackman's Occupational Therapy. 5th ed. Philadelphia: J.B. Lippincott & Co. 1978.
5. Comstock RL, Mayers RL, Folsom JC. Simple physical activities for the elderly. Hospital and Community Psychiatry 1979; 30(6): 377-380.
6. Smedley M. Model programme. Geriaction April 1980: 27-30.
7. Squires B. Reality orientation. Unpublished paper.
8. Norris AD, Abu El Eileh MTR. Reminiscence groups. Nursing Times 11 Aug. 1982; 1368-1369.
9. Squires B, Cameron J. "This is your life" book. Sydney, unpublished paper.

Further reading

Bellchamber M. Activities, games, quizzes. Pamphlet distributed by the Australian Association for Geriatric Nursing Care, Miranda, PO Box 569, NSW 2228.

Day centres: a concept worth considering, Book 3. A Project of the Returned Servicemen's League, NSW. Available from the Repatriation General Hospital, Hospital Road, Concord, NSW 2137, Australia.

Getting on . . . a handbook for older people and those who care for them. Sydney: Health Commission of New South Wales, Division of Health Promotion, 1981.

Chapter 12

Community Resources for the Aged

Objectives

To enable the reader to:

1. identify the major problems encountered when providing services for the care of aged people in the community;
2. be aware of the availability of services and how to gain access to them;
3. be able to act as adviser/advocate for those in their care who require special services;
4. appreciate the need to consider individual differences and preferences of the aged persons for whom services are to be provided;
5. understand that the provision of appropriate services depends to a large extent on adequate assessment;
6. discuss the cost of community care in terms of cost to families who care for their older member, and hopefully be slow to criticise those who choose to discontinue care in the face of family hardship;
7. be aware that the majority of old people are living in the community and either caring for themselves or being cared for by their family members, with or without some back-up services.

This chapter is concerned with resources and services which provide a system of care for the older person living in the community. Most elderly people would choose to remain in their own homes, in familiar surroundings, and it has been demonstrated that for those who are able to do so many problems, including some medical and psychological problems, can be prevented.

System of care

The vast majority of older people are physically able and have the potential support of spouse or co-resident, but for some it only becomes possible to maintain themselves in the community when a lot of time is spent by families, volunteers and services which provide personal care, meals, home nursing and linen services, transport, home maintenance and other assistance which enables them to stay at home.

The aim of any system of care should be:

- to delay for as long as possible the onset of disability;
- to promote and prolong maximum independence through the resources of family and neighbourhood, backed by the provision of appropriate services.

These services should be readily accessible when required, either for respite for carers or for long-term care when the elderly person is no longer able to remain at home.

It is interesting to note that admission to institutional care is often necessary, not because of the nature of the service or care required, but because of the difficulties associated with the increased number of times it is required and the availability, or lack, of resources and services to meet that requirement. Although mutual assistance enables many older couples to live independently despite their frailty, the illness or the onset of disability for one of the partners can lead to the institutionalisation of both if help is not available.

Overview

In most Western industrialised countries about 95 per cent of elderly people live in the community in private households, with only a small minority needing special care in institutions such as hospitals and nursing homes. The Australian Bureau of Statistics estimates that 93.6 per cent of people over the age of sixty-five live in independent households; 2.2 per cent live in hostels and retirement villages; while about 4.2 per cent occupy accommodation in nursing homes and hospitals.[1] It would seem then that, following the trend in similar societies, the majority of elderly Australians are maintained in the community.

Responsibility for provision of services

The responsibility for providing services for the care of the elderly members of the community is shared by:

- Federal, state and, to a lesser degree, local government systems;
- health and welfare departments;
- both the charitable non-government and the profit-based private sectors.

Each of these groups plays a role in what is acknowledged to be "a very large and complex yet poorly integrated service network".[2]

Many criticisms have been voiced of the fragmentation of responsibility with the consequent difficulties in co-ordination and overlap and duplication of service programs. Another major issue has been that of the imbalance between institutional and community-based care, and committees were commissioned to investigate and report on these and other issues. Two such reports were the McLeay Report in 1982 and the Richmond Report in 1984.

One of the outcomes of the McLeay Report has been the establishment of a special unit to provide the government with policy advice on all initiatives and programs which provide facilities and services for the aged.[3]

The Commonwealth Government has created The Department of Community Services and Health, while the state governments have established Offices of Care for the Aged. The Department of Community Services and Health provides a focus for funding aspects of community and long-term care for aged and disabled persons. The Offices of Care for the Aged act as focal points for the development of services in each state and also to develop a national policy on how best to provide assistance to meet the need for accommodation and home care for aged persons.

Funding of services

Funds for the provision of services will obviously be limited and this in turn leads to intense competition for available funds between those responsible for various services. It also seems likely that groups most able to identify their problems and perhaps suggest realistic options for dealing with them will have a better chance of securing funds. This would be especially true if these options came within the existing constraints on resources.

Groups such as:

- The New South Wales Council of the Ageing
- The Combined Pensioners Association
- VOTE (The Voice of the Elderly)
- Carers Association
- Social Welfare Action Group

are all examples of groups who are seeking to ensure adequate resources for community services for aged persons and those who care for them.

Demand for services

Ageing is not synonymous with ill health, but the aged do have a greater need for health services than the general population because of chronic illness, disability and frailty which increases with age. Demographers have predicted that the proportion of people in the population of Australia who are over sixty-five years of age will increase from 12.2 per cent in 1983 to 14 per cent in the year 2000, then increase rapidly to 18.6 per cent by the year 2020. The prediction for those over seventy-five years is even more dramatic. They are expected to increase from 29.7 per cent in 1983 to 38.6 per cent by the year 2000[4] (see Table 12.1).

Table 12.1 The Aged 1983 to 2020 ('000)

	Under 75 (a)		**75 and Over**			
	Number	**% of Aged**	**Number**	**% of Aged**	**Total aged**	**% of Population**
1983	1319.0	70.3	558.0	29.7	1877.0	12.2
1984	1340.2	69.8	580.1	30.2	1920.3	12.3
1985	1368.7	69.4	604.9	30.6	1973.6	12.5
1986	1396.4	68.7	635.6	31.3	2032.0	12.7
1987	1422.6	68.2	664.3	31.8	2086.9	12.9
1988	1448.8	67.7	692.6	32.3	2141.4	13.1
1989	1470.7	67.0	722.8	33.0	2193.5	13.3
1990	1490.0	66.5	751.7	33.5	2241.7	13.4
2000	1592.4	61.4	1002.8	38.6	2595.2	14.0
2010	2006.1	63.6	1150.4	36.4	3156.5	15.7
2020	2628.9	65.7	1375.3	34.3	4004.2	18.6

Source: Australia's Population Trends and Prospects 1984 (DIEA, 1984).
Note: (a) The population of pensionable age (males 65 and over and females 60 and over).

Resources

Although services are provided by government and voluntary agencies and private enterprise, most are provided by 'faceless carers'. These people are unpaid and do not appear in statistics about the cost of care in the community; it would seem that the greatest resource for the elderly person is people. These people may be family members, a kind and caring neighbour or friend, or perhaps volunteers who offer to visit or help in other ways.

The family

Studies by Kendig[5] and others have shown that the chief support available to the elderly in the community is the family and that the most immediate form of family support is from a spouse, followed by that of children if they are available. There is, however, an increasing number of widowed old people, the majority of whom are women, who are alone and without family members to support them.

Despite this situation the resourcefulness of the individual old person can be great and should not be overlooked. It is very important for those who provide care not to be overprotective and to allow as much independence as possible. If this is not allowed, then the motivation of older people to call on their own resources may be lost and lead to their dependence on available services. It may even lead to their seeking institutional care.

Finance

Another important resource is finance, and home ownership has been shown to be a major determinant of the elderly person's financial situation. It is argued by some that income support is the most important of all services and it would seem that the most important way of promoting independence is for old people to have the financial means to make choices for themselves.[6]

Financial assistance is provided by the Commonwealth Government through the Department of Social Security which is responsible for the payment of pensions to those who are eligible. These include:

- aged pension
- widow's pension

More recently granted as a result of lobbying by the Carers Association is the Carer's Pension. This is granted to those who are responsible for caring for their spouse at home.

Benefits

All these pensions carry benefits, and a study of the value of these fringe benefits to pensioners[4] (p 15) found that they are of considerable value to many pensioners and add to their standard of living.

These benefits include such things as:

- Rent Assistance .... Department of Housing.
- Funeral Benefit .... Department of Social Security.
- Domiciliary Care Benefit .... Department of Social Security.

The latter benefit is paid to those who stay at home to care for an elderly relative and is subject to certain qualifying conditions. While it greatly underprices the actual cost to the carer, it is nevertheless a welcome benefit. It is different from the Carer's Pension mentioned earlier.

Concessions

Concessions are also available to those who are in receipt of a pension. Examples of these are:

- telephone rental reduction .... Telecom.
- electricity rebate .... Electricity Commission.
- transport concessions .... Motor Transport Department.

  (Certificates are issued automatically to those who are eligible for pensions.)
- Free medical care is available and drivers' licences are issued free of charge to those in receipt of a pension.
- Rebates on current council rates and water and sewerage rates are also available and there are certain theatres, hairdressers, etc. which provide concessional rates for pensioners.

It is important to note that these benefits and concessions are not available to old people *per se,* but only to those who qualify for the payment of a pension, be it aged, widow's or invalid pension. It is also important to be aware of the financial anxieties of some older people on 'fixed incomes' and also of some families who are caring for an elderly member. More and more it is becoming necessary for wives to return to the workforce to maintain adequate family incomes in the face of inflation. If they are required to stay at home to care for ageing parents, without financial compensation, then financial stresses can result. This is not only an economic issue, however, but includes the question of social cost, which is not always easy to assess. Care should be taken not to prolong the responsibility for caring to the extent that there is a breakdown in family relationships.

Housing

Not every older person wishes to live with family or relatives, even when this option is open to them. However, they may be unable to cope with the maintenance of their own family home and the provision of alternate accommodation which is suitable to their needs becomes necessary.

Accommodation is provided by the Housing Commission while some types of special accommodation are operated by government organisations and others are privately owned or run by church or voluntary organisations. Examples of these are:

- group homes
- hostels
- retirement villages, many of which provide a three-level system of care. Unit and hostel accommodation is provided, with hospital accommodation also being available as it becomes necessary.

The Aged or Disabled Homes Act

This was enacted in 1954 to encourage the provision of suitable homes for aged or disabled persons, where they could live in conditions approaching as nearly as possible normal domestic life and, in the case of married couples, with proper regard to the companionship of husband and wife. Under this act:

- a grant towards the capital cost of a home can be made to an eligible organisation;
- provision is made for the payment of an amount in respect of each person who:
  - has attained the age of eighty years, or
  - is receiving approved personal care services, and
  - is residing in accommodation provided by the approved organisation on a prescribed date.

There is, however, a shortage of low-rent accommodation for those who require it, and many pay up to 90 per cent of their income for accommodation. The Federal Government has expressed a commitment to providing more hostel accommodation and has also introduced assessment by specially appointed teams as a prerequisite for admission to nursing homes and some government services. Because of the individual differences and preferences among the elderly population, as in any other, there needs to be maximum flexibility and a wide range of alternatives to meet the broad spectrum of needs, although hostels and houses have a valuable place in the total range of provision.

Domestic help

For many elderly people in the community the need is not for health care services or for personal care but for help with domestic chores and home maintenance.

Home Care Services are often available and attract government funding. While these services are for housekeeping and personal care, some agencies also provide home maintenance services. The importance of these services is indicated by the fact that the demand is greater than the supply.

Health care

For those who do require care there are a number of services available:

- community nursing service by nurses attached to community health centres;
- district nursing services;
- home nursing services attached to local councils;
- chiropody services – very important for the comfort and welfare of the elderly person – are available either at senior citizens centres or community health centres and in some areas home visits may be arranged;
- dental services are provided free to eligible pensioners at public hospitals, mobile dental clinics and dental hospitals;
- hearing aid service – pensioners may receive free hearing aids from the National Acoustics Laboratories;
- Extended Care Services, as proposed by the McLeay Report, are being implemented and these will comprise a range of services such as:
  - inpatient geriatric and rehabilitation units
  - multidisciplinary assessment teams
  - day hospitals, respite care, day care
  - home nursing
  - home care
  - delivered meals
  - home maintenance
  - equipment and aids
  - laundry and transport services
  - access to hostel and nursing home accommodation.

Volunteers and community services

According to Hardwick and Graycar,[7] there are about 36,967 organisations in Australia that use voluntary labour, with an estimated 1,093,895 persons involved. This represents about 10 per cent of the population providing voluntary services to those in need of them. Many of these voluntary workers are past retirement age themselves and the majority of them are women. Hardwick and Graycar state that "the extent of voluntary activity throughout Australia is such that our welfare services could not continue without the input of volunteer activity and the issue then becomes one of the degree to which we rely on volunteers for the continuation of these services". Reports such as the McLeay and Richmond reports suggest that there will be an even greater reliance on volunteers in the future because of funding deficits.

One service area which is very dependent on volunteers is Meals-on-Wheels. Unfortunately, this does not project beyond the volunteer system, with no provision being made for the delivery of meals at weekends.

Summary

The majority of elderly people live in the community and most maintain themselves, but for those who require services these should be available, accessible and, above all, appropriate to the needs of that particular individual. Those who provide services should be aware of the diversity of needs within the group of people for whom these services are provided. There is currently a much greater demand for services than previously because of the increased numbers of elderly people in the population; this will of course affect their availability and in turn their accessibility.

Nurses have a responsibility which they share with other service providers to be aware of available services and of how to gain access to them, so that they can help those in their care who may need such services. Ideally, the assessment of need should be made in consultation with others involved in caring and with the consumer, so that services are not 'imposed' by professional caregivers.

Multidisciplinary assessment which includes assessment of a person's medical, social, psychological and functional needs is seen as a means of reducing inappropriate admission to nursing homes and of referring people to appropriate services. We must also be aware that the consumer retains the right to refuse services even though we may consider that they are necessary. Older people may not even share your view of them as being old and thus refuse the services offered.

Unfortunately, community services are drastically under-resourced and rely to a large extent on volunteers who are very active and invaluable in the provision of services. Care must be taken, however, to ensure that policy planning is not based on the premise that volunteers will always be available to meet unmet needs. Care *in* the community should not become care *by* the community without adequate support from government sources. There is a further list of services at the end of this chapter.

Case study

Mrs M is 69 years old and her husband is five years older. They have three children all of whom are married with children of their own. One daughter and her family live in the next suburb, while the other daughter and son have moved interstate and see their parents about twice a year, although it was only once last year. Mrs M is well apart from a few 'arthriticy pains', but Mr M had a heart attack a few months ago and needs to 'take care'. He tires very easily and can't do much around the house any more. Since Mr M's health has been deteriorating, the family are urging their parents to sell their house and move into a retirement village, but Mr and Mrs M are unwilling to do so, stating that they want to live out their remaining days together in the house they have lived in for most of their married lives and say that they will manage.

Questions

1. What do you see as Mr and Mrs M's resources or potential resources?
2. What government assistance, rebates or benefits do you consider they may be eligible for, and what additional information would you need from them to assess their eligibility?
3. What services might be available to them to enable them to remain in their own home as they wish?

References

1. Australian Bureau of Statistics. Projections of the population of Australia. Canberra: Australian Government Publishing Service, 1981.
2. Hemer JM, Gibson DM. Provision for whom? Provision of services in health welfare and family in later life. Sydney: New South Wales Council on the Ageing, 1983.
3. In a home or at home: accommodation and home care for the aged. Report from the House of Representatives Standing Committee on Expenditure. Canberra: Australian Government Publishing Service, 1982.
4. Dixon D, Shannon P. The health and welfare dollar: will the aged get a fair share? Paper presented to the 9th Annual Conference of The NSW Council on the Ageing, Sydney, 1985.
5. Kendig HL. Community care in health welfare and family in later life. Sydney: The NSW Council on the Ageing, 1983.
6. Russell C. The ageing experience. Sydney: Allen and Unwin, 1981.
7. Hardwick J, Graycar A. Volunteers in non-government welfare organisations in Australia: a working paper. Social Welfare Research Centre, University of New South Wales, Reports and Proceedings, No. 25, 1982.

Further reading

Banks G. Options: a handbook for the elderly and those who care for them. Melbourne: Dove Communications, 1984.

Care of the elderly: Current issues and future prospects. Proceedings of the 19th Annual Conference of Australian Gerontology, Sydney, 1984.

Ford B. The elderly Australian. Victoria: Penguin Books, 1984.

Howe A, ed. Towards an older Australia. Queensland: University of Queensland Press, 1981.

Resources

Where to obtain information about services for the aged

★ ★ ★ The Combined Pensioners Association has prepared a directory of services for aged persons in various municipalities.

★ ★ ★ The NSW Council on the Ageing has also compiled a document called *Services for The Aged in NSW.*

★ ★ ★ *Ninety Steps: A Simple Guide to Government, Fringe and other Community Benefits for the Aged in NSW* is also available from The Council on The Ageing.

★ ★ ★ The following Federal Government departments will provide information:
Department of Social Security
Department of Veterans Affairs
Department of Education, Employment and Training
Department of Community Services and Health
Housing Commission

★★★ State Government departments:
NSW: Department of Youth and Community Services
SA and Tasmania: Department of Community Welfare
Victoria and WA: Department of Community Services
Queensland: Department of Family Services
NT: Department of Health and Community Development
ACT: Welfare Branch of Department of Territories

★★★ In many suburbs there are Community Information Centres which provide valuable information regarding activities as well as services for the aged.

Emergencies

★★★ Financial and material assistance is available through The Department of Community Services and Health.

★★★ Voluntary agencies provide short-term emergency assistance in the form of food orders, clothing, finance, accommodation, transport and companionship.

Chapter 13

Loss and Grief in the Elderly

Objectives

To enable the reader to:

1. define the terms 'loss', 'bereavement' and 'grief';
2. explain the concept of loss;
3. identify the factors which influence an elderly person's response to loss;
4. categorise the types of losses experienced by the elderly person;
5. describe the manifestations of grief in elderly people;
6. identify the needs of the bereaved;
7. describe the types of supportive behaviour in the nurse which will provide comfort and aid in the resolution of grief;
8. describe the bases of the attitudes nurses and elderly people have about dying and death;
9. identify the needs of the dying elderly person;
10. discuss the principles of care of the dying elderly person;
11. identify the needs of the nurse while caring for bereaved and dying elderly people;
12. suggest methods by which the nurse can meet the identified needs.

It is not possible to live without experiencing loss, grief and the process of dying. In this chapter it is proposed to discuss:

- the various types of losses that the elderly are likely to experience;
- the pattern of responses that are typically manifested as a result;
- the nature of the process of dying in the elderly;
- the nurse's responsibilities in bringing about an effective resolution to the above physical, emotional and social crises.

Definitions

Loss refers to the usually forced 'giving up a valued internal or external support that is required to meet basic needs, such as a person, thing, relationship, situation, status, role, ritual, health or independence'.[1] The person, therefore, feels bereft of something very significant to his physical, emotional, social or spiritual well-being. Some of the basic needs which may not be met, at least in the short term, are companionship, love, security, ambition and self-esteem.

Grief is a very subjective response to a loss. It is what the affected person feels about that loss. The experience of grief is a very personal thing which cannot be seen or quantified by an observer. Grief is characterised by a sequence of emotional and physical states,[2] all of which have social consequences for the survivor.

Bereavement is an objective, socially prescribed state of being in society following the loss or death of a person with close ties to the survivor. It in no way describes the survivor's response to the loss or death. When a husband dies, his wife who survives him is said to be bereaved. In this instance, grief is the response the survivor has to her bereavement.[3]

The aged are no strangers to loss and grief. Golda Meier, a former Israeli Prime Minister, is quoted as saying: 'Being seventy is no crime . . . but it is no joke either'.[4] What prompted her comment is not explained but it could be speculated that there were two basic reasons: first, that the longer people live, the more likely they are to have experienced many losses and therefore griefs; and, second, as people age the inevitability of their own death quite obviously draws closer.

Whether this speculation is justified or not, it defines two facets of life facing all human beings, particularly the elderly. Not only does a longer period of life intensify the potential for them to experience more losses, but it is also likely to increase the frequency with which these losses occur.

The kinds of losses that may have to be faced are many – physical, psychosocial, occupational, financial, cultural and environmental.[5,6]

A number of writers have suggested that, although various attitudes towards death have been identified among the elderly, generally speaking, their attitudes towards death are different from those of younger dying persons.[7-9]

Kinds of losses experienced by the aged

There are many kinds of losses which the elderly experience, including loss of body functions and relationships, and other more intangible factors such as self-esteem.

Loss of body functions

As a consequence of the ageing process various impairments of body functions become apparent.

Sensory losses are very common in the aged, particularly loss of hearing and of vision.[10] Both losses require the person to make adjustments to his life cycle. He has to accept reduced contacts with the sights and sounds of his world and concurrently an increased dependence on medical services for surgical interventions, spectacles and hearing aids.

Not uncommonly, loss of hearing seems to bring about a change in personality functioning.[11] The person afflicted is more likely to become irritable with 'contraptions that don't work' or 'batteries that are always running down'. Difficulty in hearing conversations may result in the person becoming depressed and suspicious about other people's intentions.[5] His resultant behaviour may be interpreted as deliberately difficult and unreasonable, so leading to his avoidance by others.

The frustration experienced by speakers unable to make themselves understood by the hearing impaired person results in their speaking more slowly and loudly. The speech may often become 'telegraphic', much like that characteristic of a two-year-old child. So, not only does the elderly person have to adjust to being unable to hear, in addition he is likely to be subjected to a less-than-adult type of conversation. The resultant attitude created in the speaker who cannot make himself readily understood may then be transferred to other interactions with that or other aged persons similarly afflicted. Simply as a consequence of a hearing loss, the aged person may find himself being treated as a child in more ways than one. Nurses must take care not to fall into the trap of believing that being deaf is synonymous with having greatly reduced mental facilities.

Elderly people with vision and hearing deficits develop a greater reliance on touch for comfort and pleasure. Dangott and Kalish[6] refer to this as being 'touch hungry'. Given that old people are already deprived of physical contact,[12] those with a marked sensory loss are in even greater need of genuine affection – a touch, a hug or a kiss from those who care for them.

Loss of sexual function is invariably associated with ageing. Dangott and Kalish[6] believe that this and sensory losses 'can be the most personally devitalizing and annihilating of all' (p 133). Sexual feelings, expression and intimacies contribute very much to a sense of self.[6] As sexual function diminishes, part of the self dies. The process may be gradual or sudden, depending upon such factors as sex, physiological changes, illness, opportunity for relationships, personal expectations and societal attitudes. Studies have shown that reduced sexual activity between couples is likely, in men, to be due to reduced physical ability and a change in attitudes and, in women, to a lack of opportunity and maybe interest.[13,14]

Some elderly may be subliminally influenced by 'sexual ageism'. Hall *et al*[15] define this as being the 'social expectation that the aged do not have and should not have sexual relationships' (p 29). However, other authors suggest that many aged people retain a healthy interest in sex; they retain sexual desires and continue to be sexually active when the opportunity arises.[17]

For those whose reduced physiological abilities or lack of opportunity make sexual pleasures and excitement something associated only with their younger days, sadness and depression may result. These feelings may further reduce the person's ability to function sexually and increase the resentment at 'missing out'.

Nurses should be aware and accepting of the elderly person's sexual needs for what they are, and not belittle them or consider them in any way abnormal. Encouragement and opportunities for such activities as body massaging may meet at least some of the aged person's sexual needs. Thought should be given by staff in retirement and nursing homes to ensuring that elderly couples are given adequate privacy.

Loss of fertility is a source of grief more likely to be of concern to women because they are the child-bearers. This role is brought to an abrupt and obvious end by the occurrence of the menopause. There is no equivalent naturally occurring sudden loss of fertility in men. In a society that values youth, beauty and sexuality, the post-menopausal and ageing woman may feel her attractiveness to men and usefulness to society has vanished. For the woman who has never had children, the onset of menopause signifies the end to any dreams she may have retained of bearing children. Her response may be a combination of anger, resentment, regret, sadness and depression.[5]

Eena Job[17] found that parenthood had been a central experience in many aged people's lives. For these people, adjustment to loss of fertility may occur more readily when they can enter into the joys, pleasures and concerns of being grandparents.

Loss of mobility frequently occurs in the elderly because of arthritis. Pain almost inevitably accompanies attempts to move degenerating joints. Consequently, the affected person may find it increasingly difficult to go shopping or clean the house, and even preparing meals may become an impossibility. Of necessity, aged persons are forced to depend on others to help them with even the ordinary activities of daily living.

Mobility may also be hampered as a result of a cerebrovascular accident, fracture, peripheral vascular disease, amputation or neurological disorders.

Whatever the cause of the loss of mobility it, plus the accompanying loss of independence, may produce a very great sense of loss.[5] Irritability, resentment, demanding behaviour and constant criticism of all attempts to meet the person's demands may be manifestations of the intense grief and frustration being felt. Understanding, patience and gentle encouragement by the nurse are required in these circumstances. The person should be given opportunities to make choices and take control of his care as far as is possible.

Loss of other body functions can also occur. They may be related to any of the body systems – digestive, cardiac, respiratory, urinary, endocrine and neurological. Regardless of how the impairment of functions is manifest, the overall effect on the aged person is to reinforce for him the fact that his health is not what it was. Some grieve over the loss of physical well-being. Others accept the changes and are therefore able to make appropriate adjustments.

Nursing staff should be aware of the various impairments of body functions which might be amenable to medical intervention. For example, sudden stress incontinence is a particularly embarrassing problem endured by a number of older women. It can be a source of great shame and distress and be responsible for an unwillingness on their part to go out or socialise.

Loss of relationships

Just as the elderly experience changes in their physical condition, so too are there changes in their relationships with people. In psychological terms this occurrence is called disengagement. It is described as being 'a process in which many of the relationships between an older person and members of his social groups are relinquished and others attenuated so that there is a mutual withdrawal'.[5(p 207)] Not only is there a reduction in the number of social contacts an aged person has, but the nature of the relationships is also likely to change.

Kinship relationships

Death of a spouse is a highly significant loss for an aged person. A couple may have spent fifty or more years together. The Toowong study[17] found that certainly not all long marriages were of the 'Darby and Joan' type. Some had endured more with trust and respect than great happiness. Consequently, a certain easiness and maybe tolerance is likely to develop between the marriage partners as they become accustomed to each other's ways and foibles. The incapacitation or death of one partner, therefore, can cause great grief to the survivor who has to adjust, late in life, to a whole new set of circumstances including reduced social contacts and increased isolation, loneliness and loss of affection, particularly physical affection. Financial and other decisions previously made by the deceased spouse suddenly become the responsibility of the survivor, who may lack knowledge and experience in such matters. The bereaved may be forced to move to a different abode, devoid of memories of the many activities the two once shared.

Few widows over sixty-five are likely to remarry.[5] One of the reasons for this is the non-availability of men of similar age because of their lower life expectancy. Not much is known about the reactions of the elderly to the loss of a spouse because most studies have concentrated on younger widows. Raphael[5] suggests that the elderly widow's grief reaction may be a diffuse one, manifesting itself in 'weeping, agitation and care-eliciting behaviour' (p 213). In contrast, widowers 'show angry withdrawal' (p 313). However, both elderly widows and widowers have reported 'significantly more recently developed or worsened illnesses, greater use of medication' and poor general health two months after the loss of a spouse.[18]

Both widows and widowers may demonstrate a helplessness in day-to-day activities, asking others to take over the reins and make their decisions for them. Almost 30 per cent will become depressed, particularly if they do not receive consistent and regular family support.[5] The period of time following the death of the spouse may be ritually marked off each day by the survivor, even years later. Some continue the relationship 'in fantasy or in behaviour'.[5(p 313)] As one woman put it: 'I talk to him every morning. I never make a decision without just talking it over with Max.' Her home was full of memorabilia – his clothes, his hat, his chair, his mug, photos, records. Even fingermarks he made on the bedroom wall when ataxic during his final days have been preserved.

Three intervening factors contribute to the extent to which the surviving spouse adapts to bereavement: supportive social networks, concurrent losses, and coping skills.[19] These will now be discussed in more detail.

Supportive network. This is defined by Walker *et al* (1977) as 'that set of personal contacts through which the individual maintains his/her social identity and receives emotional support, material aid and services, information and new social contacts'[19(p 466)] To help the bereaved person to reintegrate into a social group, supports must not only be available, but they must be appropriate. The nature of the assistance required by the bereaved person immediately after the spouse has died will be different from that required a month, two months or twelve months later; as Gallagher *et al* point out: 'The grief experienced at the time of the funeral has aspects that are independent from grief experienced at eight weeks post-bereavement'.[19(p 579)]

Concurrent losses. As mentioned previously, there is a likelihood that the elderly will experience an onslaught of bereavements and other losses. There may be no time to complete grieving for one loss before another occurs. Kastenbaum[3] calls this accumulation of losses in the aged 'bereavement overload'. Adaptation to so many losses is made even more difficult by the fact that there are few or no substitutes for what has been lost. It is too late to remarry, have more children, or get another job.

Coping skills are required by the bereaved person to make the adjustments necessary to live again as a single person, after so much time, with all that is entailed emotionally, socially and economically. Those that have successfully resolved maturational crises earlier in life may be better equipped emotionally, cognitively and behaviourally to meet these new crises.[19]

Loss of parents. The parents of many elderly people will have died before they themselves can be classifed as elderly. However, as life expectancy rates increase, it has certainly become possible for some parents not to die until their children become young-old. Horowitz *et al*[5] found that, regardless of how old a person was when his/her parents died, or whether the death was anticipated or not, it still resulted in a significant amount of 'symptomatic stress', particularly for unmarried women.

Loss of children may occur simply as a stage in the life cycle when grown children leave the family home. As a consequence, particularly the mother's role and responsibilities in the home are changed and, it could even be argued, in some ways diminished. The extent to which parents adjust to their 'empty nest' situation will depend on the extent to which the child's departure was 'expected or unexpected, timely or untimely, and the ambivalence and/or dependence of the relationships with the child'.[5(p 308)] Irrespective of this, most parents will experience a sense of loss and grief. There is a likelihood that their reactions will be exacerbated if most of the parents' activities and marriage have depended upon the child's presence. Lone parents without supports are probably at even more risk of being unable to resolve their loss satisfactorily.

Adult children may also be lost by premature death. The inevitable response is: 'I always expected to go first.' The parents may feel guilty that their lives have been preserved, angry that their child's life has been cut short and bewildered by why it has happened to them. The parents' grief response may be extreme when the death has occurred suddenly, or when the child was particularly 'precious' – the child they never thought they would conceive, the only child, the child there is no hope of replacing. Resolution of such grief may be protracted and unsatisfactory, particularly if relatives and friends shun references to the dead child.

Loss of a pet also produces marked grief. It is essential that the nurse does not downgrade the extent of such grief. One young-old woman's recovery from a curable illness was in serious jeopardy until her extreme agitation and concern about her dog was alleviated. A nurse was able to ascertain that the dog was being fed and cared for by a kindly neighbour. To reassure the woman even more, she had the neighbour bring the dog to the hospital. The pet may have been the aged person's only or chief source of love, particularly unconditional love. It may have belonged to a special person now gone, or it may have been acquired as a replacement for a lost partner or child.[5]

Social losses

Loss of friends and peers happens with monotonous regularity to the elderly person. Many ritually scan the 'Deaths' column in the daily papers. Each year the continuing decrease in the number of Christmas cards received is further evidence for the aged person that more and more peers are dying. It can reach the stage where the old person is saying: 'I'm the only one left from my group now.'

The loss of friends may occur as a consequence of geographical separation brought about by changing family circumstances, health or interests. Whatever the reason for the moving away of long-term friends, elderly people can find themselves devoid of peer company – especially men, because of their shorter life expectancy. Feelings of loneliness or sadness may overwhelm the survivors to the point that they begin to hope they will soon follow in the footsteps of those who have gone before.

Nothing can be done to stop the death of the elderly person's friends. What can be done, however, is the development of community awareness schemes so that contact can be maintained with the person and new acquaintances gradually and periodically established.

Loss of work, and retirement, are covered more fully elsewhere in this book. However, it needs to be discussed here, too, because of the magnitude of the consequences of such a loss on the rest of the person's life. In Australia it has been customary for most people to retire between sixty and sixty-five years of age. The economic recession has forced some employers to retrench workers, often with little warning. In one fell swoop, many people have lost not only their job, but a purposeful daily routine, workmates, an income and a clearly designated role in society.[6]

Even those who have had time to anticipate their impending retirement experience the same losses. The difference is that they at least have had the opportunity to get used to the idea and plan for their retirement.[21] Some retirees have skills and knowledge that can be utilised in part-time consulting work. They are able to ease into the retirement role. For the majority of workers in our society employment ceases on a particular day forever. These are the people for whom the days thereafter can drift on into years of aimlessness and boredom unless they can quickly establish new goals and relationships for themselves. Rowles[22] describes the situation of 'Stan' whose 'one source of enrichment was provided by his friendship network' (p 11) at work. The friends lived in different parts of the city so that after he retired he was rarely able to meet with them again. On the occasions when they did meet, he found they no longer had anything in common to talk about.

For the woman who has not had employment outside the home and whose time has been taken up with domestic and 'extracurricular' activities, the sudden continued presence of her husband in the home can be a definite source of irritation. 'He gets in the way and always wants me either to be doing something for or with him.' The husband, on the other hand, has to devise things to do to occupy the days once taken up with his work. He can feel at a loss in his own home. The wife seems to have much to fill her days, while he is bored. He may resent the time she spends on out-of-the-house activities, from which he is excluded. Each day has become a whole new ball game for the two of them. One very successful artisan became so disenchanted with the retirement situation at home that he reopened his studio!

Another change associated with retirement is a drop in income[21] which may only become a problem if there are unexpected expenses, such as hospital bills or major car repairs. For the man who unexpectedly loses his job, the loss of income may force the abandonment of certain leisure and social activities. Initially he may become apathetic, depressed, ashamed, withdrawn and helpless. If unresolved, his grief may become chronic, characterised by bitterness, anger, depression and helplessness. Some may develop psychosomatic ailments. Others may attempt to drown their despair and plummeting self-esteem in alcohol. It is thought that such people have a high morbidity risk, though to date no systematic studies have been done to confirm this.[5]

Loss of roles occurs in conjunction with all the previously mentioned losses. Death of a significant person, loss of employment and impairment of body functions all bring about changes in the bereaved person's status 'which involves a shift in social roles'.[5]

What was expected by society from the wife, the able-bodied person and the worker is not what is expected from the widow, disabled or unemployed person. Because people's friendships are attached to their roles, any role loss can reduce their opportunities to participate socially. With reduced social resources, elderly people's susceptibility to stress is increased and they are more likely to become dependent, isolated and to experience poorer health. Resocialisation and adjustment to the newly prescribed social identity is likely to occur more easily in those persons with less role loss, who are younger and who have greater personal resources.[23]

One of the goals of the 'death education' and 'loss and grief courses currently being developed is to try to expand the personal resources of the bereaved person. The information given aims to put people in a better position to make use of available community resources and to make informed decisions about a whole range of matters – wills, funeral procedures, finances, legal aid and so on. Such information may be of more value to the bereaved elderly woman, who will find herself in a world of aged women run primarily by younger men.

Intangible losses

These losses are usually closely associated with the body function and relationship losses already discussed. The fact that they tend to occur as a consequence of the more concrete types of losses in no way means that they are of secondary importance to the elderly sufferers. Loss of motivation, ambition, confidence, the opportunity to choose, privacy, personal freedom, independence, self-esteem, faith and hope are examples of intangible losses.[12]

The aged woman with stress incontinence will quickly lose her confidence after experiencing the embarrassment of having urine run down her legs while in a social situation. The naked old gentleman being washed in an unscreened bed by a young female nurse will soon get the idea he is not valued as an individual with rights. An eminent eighty-year-old Australian scientist, when being interviewed on television recently, said he found his newly developed loss of motivation to complete already begun projects a very distressing and frustrating change.

The tendency for some nurses and others to dictate to elderly residents what they should eat and wear, when they should get up, have a bath or go to bed, does nothing for their self-esteem. Elderly people have a life-time of experiences behind them, and nurses must foster in their approach to the elderly a genuine interest in unearthing their accomplishments. The resultant admiration may do much to bolster fragile self-esteem and flagging spirits.

Manifestations of grief

Grief is a person's reaction to loss. 'It is a process, not a state.'[24(p 21)] The grieving process comprises a series of phases[5] which can extend over a considerable period of time. Time alone, however, does not ensure the satisfactory resolution of grief.[20] Bowlby[21] described five phases of grief and mourning. Engel, in 1962, suggested there were three phases. The different opinions serve to emphasise the fact that the phases are not clear-cut and that individual responses to loss can vary greatly.

Shock, numbness and disbelief

When a person becomes aware of a loss, the first response is stunned numbness and disbelief as he seems unable to comprehend what has happened. The response may be one of calm detachment, during which time the ego has time to muster its resources.[5] A young man described how he quite unemotionally watched his arm being devoured from his hand upwards by the rollers of a machine. Some people respond as though it was a bad dream from which they will soon wake unscathed. Others look and feel as though they have been kicked in the midriff by a horse, especially if the loss is gross and totally unexpected. This phase may last hours or days, depending on the time it takes the person to accept the reality of his loss.

When the loss is by death, Raphael[5] identifies four factors which help the bereaved face the reality of death. 'The need for the bereaved to communicate about the death to significant others; the legal processes concerned with the death such as certification; the need to arrange for the disposal of the body; and the presence and words of others who acknowledge the death' (p 34).

Two factors are particularly important in the subsequent consolidation of the reality: viewing the body, and arranging and taking part in the funeral. Many people consider it unwise, even macabre, for the bereaved to view and spend time with the body. The evidence is to the contrary.[5] A young, adopted daughter who had not seen her 87-year-old father for some months stood by the coffin looking at his pale, cold face. She noted the biopsy scar on his neck and the weariness in his emaciated face. She talked about the course his illness had taken. She cried, was silent for a time, then commented: 'You know, I think he'd think it was real great to be dressed up like that.' Her aunt laughed quietly with her. Then the daughter spoke of the times they had had together. With a final sad 'goodbye' they left to participate with the other mourners in his funeral. Later, they grouped to share over coffee their sadness and memories of a much loved and respected old man.

Developing awareness

During the second phase of the grief response, the person's emotional awareness of the reality of the loss gradually catches up with his intellectual acknowledgement of the reality. The person experiences waves of anguish which can be quite unexpectedly triggered by a particular daily occurrence or memento. They can occur with great intensity, the person crumbling in deep emotional pain and hurt. He yearns for a return to his pre-bereavement situation. A great deal of energy may be expended trying actively to will the return of what has been lost. The person may cry and feel intensely sad, anxious and helpless.[5]

Periodically, what appears to the observer as irrational anger may be expressed about the carers. An example is the adopted daughter's charge that her father (at eighty-seven years) 'could have lived much longer' if the doctor had recognised his signs and symptoms of a year ago for what they apparently were and had acted appropriately upon them. Anger may also be directed towards the deceased for being so inconsiderate and unfeeling as to die. Sometimes guilt feelings are expressed by the bereaved person, guilt that maybe he contributed to or even caused the death. This is especially likely to be so if the couple had had an ambivalent or strained relationship.

Somatic manifestations of distress usually occur concurrently with the emotional reactions. They may include palpitations, shortness of breath, sighing respirations and feelings of tightness in the throat, emptiness in the pit of the stomach and muscle weakness. Individuals are often agitated, restless and non-productively overactive; they may have difficulty initiating and carrying out the activities of daily living.[20]

The phase of developing awareness may last for months or years. It is a wearing time for the grieving person and is often exacerbated by the impatience of friends and relatives who urge him 'to get over it'.

Resolution

There comes a time when the person is able to accept the finality of his loss. The acceptance may come about quite quickly or occur gradually over several months. It involves the painful process of 'relinquishing the bonds of the relationship'[5(p 43)] and rebuilding the psychic self without the lost object. The pain of the loss has become less intense and the person is able to go on purposefully living his life while retaining a realistic memory of what has been lost.[20]

Major variations in grief

The phases and emotional and physiological reactions described above typify so-called 'normal' grief. Averill[19] described five other variations of grief. These were:

- exaggerated grief – which is abnormally intense and prolonged grief;
- abbreviated grief – grief which is short-lived, due to the immediate and appropriate replacement of the lost object, or because the loss was not a significant one;
- inhibited grief – which occurs when a person shows few signs of normal grief, but complains instead of various somatic problems;
- anticipatory grief – grief which results in anticipation of someone's death and may be abbreviated when the loss occurs;
- delayed grief – grief may be delayed for up to years if work, family or other responsibilities occupy the bereaved person's time.

Factors influencing the outcome of bereavement

Parkes[24] lists a number of antecedent, concurrent and subsequent determinants of the outcome of bereavement in general. It can be presumed that only some of these determinants will have relevance to the elderly person's reactions, because little research has been done on the subject.

Antecedent determinants

- Type of death – the cause, timeliness and predictability of the death can influence the outcome. Some elderly, for example, are more distressed by painful and protracted dying of their beloved.
- Nature of the pre-existing relationship – for those who have had either an intense, dependent or ambivalent relationship with the dead person, the mourning is more complex.[5]

- Previous losses – unresolved losses in early life and the presence of 'bereavement overload' (as discussed earlier) will increase the possibility of poor resolution of the most recent loss.

Concurrent determinants

- Sex – it is reported that women resolve grief less well than men. This may be because 'she is generally an older person in our youth-dominated society; she is single in a couple-oriented society; she is female in a male-dominated society; and she is often poor in a very affluent society'.[25(p 139)]
- Age – bereavement, particularly in the elderly, means that many adjustments have to be made in an environment often devoid of supports. Consequently, the risks of poor resolution of their grief is markedly increased.
- Personality – Parkes[24] considers some people are more 'grief-prone' than others. Inhibition of feelings is also a personality factor contributing to poor resolution of grief. It is suggested that the elderly are more likely to manifest grief through somatic symptoms than emotionally.[20,24]

Subsequent determinants

These include such things as the presence and extent of a support network, the number of secondary stresses on the bereaved person, and the variety of options available to him as he sets about reorganising his life.[24] Heyman[26] believed that the large number of female role models among the aged population made subsequent adjustment easier for widows.

Obviously there are many other factors which may influence an elderly person's adjustment to bereavement. These include genetic factors, occupation, cultural expectations and religious beliefs. A knowledge of the bereaved person's health and social history may enable the nurse to respond more sensitively to his needs and expressions of grief.

The nurse and grief

Before the nurse can be of any comfort to grieving individuals it is necessary for her to get in touch with and explore her own feelings about, and reactions to, death and any personal losses she may have experienced. Unless she does this the nurse is likely to avoid bereaved people, either physically or emotionally.

Listening and responding to bereaved people is an emotionally involving and draining experience. There will be occasions when the nurse feels quite useless and helpless in the face of someone's overwhelming grief. Following such an experience the nurse may benefit from sharing her thoughts and feelings about it with a warm and receptive person. Many hospitals, nursing homes and community nursing services do not have an established back-up system for nurses caring for bereaved people. Traditionally nurses have had to rely on informal friendship networks for any support they needed, a not always satisfactory arrangement.

Caring for the bereaved

When caring for a bereaved person, the nurse's role is essentially one of 'being' rather than 'doing'. There are no magic words the nurse can say or potions she can give to a grieving person to take away the pain. Sedatives are actually contraindicated because they serve only to postpone or permanently inhibit the grieving process.

During the initial phase of the grieving process bereaved persons need comfort and consolation.[5] Very often they desire to be held firmly, arms encircled protectively and caringly around them. This may well be an action that younger nurses especially find difficult to carry out because of being repulsed by the physically deteriorated condition of the aged person.[12] For the nurse who is reluctant to, or senses that it is inappropriate to touch the bereaved person, her quiet and continued presence will demonstrate her compassion.[5] If it is necessary for the nurse to leave the person, she should first arrange for someone to take her place so that the bereaved person is not left alone for long periods.

The nurse may be asked to provide information about the deceased's last moments or how he died. She should give the essential facts simply and concretely, being prepared to repeat them several times if the person's detached state militates against his comprehension or acceptance of them.

The nurse should not try to subdue expressions of grief. She should quietly accept displays of emotion while at the same time acknowledging how devastated the survivor must feel. To help the bereaved person accept the reality and finality of the situation, it is important that he sees the body of the deceased. The nurse should suggest to him that such an action is likely to facilitate his grieving and subsequent adjustment and then make the necessary arrangements. Only nurses working in the community are likely to see bereaved people in the second phase of their grieving.

The bereaved obviously constitute quite a small proportion of the nurse's case load in terms of numbers, but a larger proportion in terms of the contact hours they require. As a result, there may be a tendency for the nurse to bypass the bereaved person's less concrete needs in favour of those with more quickly and easily met needs.

Nursing goals of care

The nurse, as a caregiver, should have five main goals of care for the bereaved during the second phase of the grieving process. These are:

- to facilitate the emotional release;
- to assist the bereaved in recognising and expressing their yearning for the lost person;
- to facilitate reality testing by a review of death and its meaning;
- to provide other social support;
- and to initiate the basis for an ongoing caring relationship should this be needed.[5(p 358)]

Commonly, nurses have the privilege of being able to visit clients' homes. As an 'invited guest', the nurse relinquishes to the client much of her authority and control of the meeting which she could have exercised on her home territory at the health centre. However, her role as a nurse implies she has a degree of expertise and caring concern for the client. The resultant milieu, in conjunction with support and understanding acceptance by the nurse, should facilitate the expression of emotions by the bereaved person.

His home is where he will have most memories and memorabilia of the deceased. It is here that he is more likely to begin expressing his real feelings about his loss – despair, emptiness, longing, hurt, anger, and the nurse should be willing and able to respond to those feelings without shame or embarrassment. She can assure him that the various somatic and psychic phenomena he is experiencing are part of the grief response and not, as he fears, indicative of impending insanity. As the bereaved reminisces about the good and bad of the person he knew and their times together, the finality of his loss gradually becomes a reality.

Some people have beliefs which do not allow them to recognise grief as a normal and expected response to a loss. A woman weeping at the funeral of her husband killed in an accident was admonished, then exhorted, by a close friend to 'be joyful because he is now with God'. Indeed her friend did herself appear to be joyous. In these sorts of family and social situations the nurse may, without being critical of a person's beliefs, be able to explain the nature of the grief response and suggest ways in which the friends and relations can support the bereaved. The nurse can suggest and arrange for significant people such as the bereaved person's doctor and minister of religion to visit as needed. The bereaved do appreciate the visits and expressions of sympathy to them by others.[24] It reinforces for them that the dead person has been valued and was worth all the suffering they are now experiencing. In addition, it gives them more opportunities to express their feelings and talk about the deceased.

Further support

There are other community supports that it may be appropriate at some time for the nurse to mobilise. For the younger-aged person, 'Parents Without Partners' may provide an opportunity to meet people who have experienced similar losses and feelings. Sometimes support groups are established for bereaved elderly people. There is some evidence that such a group is a useful forum for older people to share feelings about coping with loss.[27] The nurse may be able to introduce the bereaved person to one or two members of other groups, such as church or senior citizens.

Pet ownership has been 'associated with an increase in social behaviour and decrease in loneliness and depression among the elderly'.[28(p 9)] However, the nurse should be aware that, at a time of loss, 'the burden of caring for a pet may become overwhelming to the elderly'.[28(p 8)] She may need to organise for a relative or neighbour to take care of it temporarily. Other forms of practical assistance may be required, for example, ensuring the bereaved can get to the cemetery, negotiating the bureaucratic maze of the Social Security Department, and helping with income tax returns.

By bringing about the bereaved person's reintegration into the social group the nurse is at the same time increasing the client's self-esteem, the basis of psychological health.[29] The nurse may further promote the bereaved elderly person's self-esteem by fostering his independence. As the resolution of his loss progresses, the nurse should change the nature and reduce the extent of her support. Gradually, he will be expected to make decisions again, utilise his capabilities and take control of his life. With confidence and self-esteem returning, the bereaved person can once again derive some satisfaction from his daily interactions and activities.

The final loss: death of the self

The longer a person lives, the nearer he comes to the day he will die. Reminders of his finiteness come from within his body. There is no escaping the reality – death is a certainty. By looking back over his life the individual can evaluate where he fitted into the scheme of things. He has come full circle and acceptance of that fact is the last developmental task to be mastered.[5,21]

Attitudes of the elderly to dying and death

Death means different things to different people of different ages in different cultures. For some it simply means 'the end'. Wass *et al*[30] found this view to be more common among urban elderly whereas rural elderly inclined to believe in an afterlife. Death may be thought of as a punishment by some, as a reward by others, and as the unknown by a few.

The behavioural characteristics of elderly people facing death have also been found to vary. Birren[9] grouped people into Welcomers, Accepters, Postponers, Disdainers and Fearers. In the Toowong (Brisbane) study, one-quarter of the sample were classified as death-postponers, and one-tenth death-deniers. The one-fifth who were death-welcomers were not often depressed, but just 'ready to go'. A high proportion of them came from the lower socioeconomic class. Keith[31] also found low-income people tended to look forward to death.

More than half the Toowong respondents were classified as death-accepters. They believed death to be 'their natural destiny'.[17] Kalish and Reynolds[6] also found that older people were less afraid of death and, not surprisingly, that they think more about it.

For a small minority of elderly people, death may be seen as a better alternative to a life without meaning.[21] The elderly who do fear death are more likely to be the unfortunate ones who have become disengaged from social interaction[32] or who moved away from their home and community and were relocated in nursing homes or other institutions.[1]

What does concern most elderly people, however, is the process of dying. They fear prolonged illness, dependency, pain, rejection, isolation,[33] immobility and loss of control over their bodies.[34] It has been found that almost half dying old patients are fully conscious and in contact with reality until the moment of death[3] so it would seem that, for the sick elderly, their fears of experiencing at least some loss of control over their bodies is quite justified.

Needs of the dying elderly person

The dying aged have many needs – physical, psychological, social and spiritual. Their needs are not any less simply because they are older, maybe less active and less involved in the wider world. Rather their needs vary, not only between people, but within the one person at different times, just as they do with younger people. It is imperative, then, that the nurse does not stereotype what she considers to be the person's needs. She should be prepared to ask the needs of every individual in her care, listen to their replies and act appropriately on them.

For an elderly person, death of the self has an inevitability and closeness about it. The anticipation of this loss may cause a grief-like reaction (sadness, anxiety and depression). As a consequence, the needs of the elderly dying person closely match those of bereaved persons. They are therefore likely to benefit from opportunities to discuss their feelings about the dying process and death.

The dying elderly also have a need to reminisce and, more specifically, to totally review their lives. Reminiscence, 'the act, process or fact of recalling the past',[35(p 266)] is regarded by many carers of the elderly to be a way of avoiding the often not so pleasant realities of the present and the future. Butler[35] considers that reminiscence has a purpose, particularly those aspects of it relating to the 'life review'. He sees the life review 'as a naturally occurring universal mental process characterized by the progressive return to consciousness of past experiences and, particularly, the resurgence of unresolved conflicts; simultaneously, and normally, these revived experiences and conflicts are surveyed and reintegrated'.[35(p 266)]

The life review process is not confined to the elderly. It frequently occurs in terminally ill people and those in crisis. In reviewing his life the elderly person takes stock of what he has achieved, where he has failed and of what remains unaccomplished or unresolved. By exposing and reorganising the past, the person gains a more complete picture of the self and its purpose in life. Paradoxically, the result is frequently the dignified acceptance by the person of his approaching death. In addition, a study by Matthieu[4] found that 40 per cent of his sample gained most comfort and support from 'memories of a full life', ahead of their 'religion' (30 per cent) and 'love from those around me' (25 per cent).

Not all people have a satisfactory outcome to their life review. Some will consider their life a failure, others will have very real grief about dastardly deeds they have done. It is these people who make a significant contribution to the increased suicide rate found in old age.[35]

The nurse's role in the care of the dying elderly person

Discussion here will be confined to the care of the 'normally' dying elderly person. The palliative care of an aged person in the terminal phase of a progressive illness is considered to be outside the scope of this chapter.

The qualities and skills a nurse requires in order to relate to and care for the elderly dying person are similar to those necessary to comfort and support the bereaved. One of these skills is the ability to listen. Young nurses may find that, in the presence of a garrulous and reminiscing old person, this skill deserts them. The significance of the life review, therefore, and the elderly person's behaviour is lost to them.[35]

Other difficulties may also be encountered by nurses caring for elderly dying people. The nurse's concept of and attitudes towards death may be quite different from those of the elderly, particularly if there is a large age discrepancy between the two. The young tend to view death with awe and as a tragedy. As indicated earlier, most elderly people are not afraid of death. So the nurse and her client 'are operating and reacting from two very different frames of reference'.[9(p 214)] As a result, the nurse may be insensitive to, and therefore unable to meet, some of the needs of her client. Age differences may also lead to a failure in communication.[9] The nurse's relative lack of experience in interpreting verbal and non-verbal cues may lead to a misinterpretation of the elderly person's needs. In contrast, the elderly are usually skilled in 'reading between the lines'. They will quickly perceive if the young nurse is reluctant to talk about what they would like to talk about – death. As a consequence, another of the elderly dying person's needs goes unmet.

A problem which has long been recognised in acute care hospitals has been shown to exist also in institutions for the elderly. In general hospitals nurses categorise patients as either 'good' or 'bad'.[36] In nursing homes the usual good/bad dichotomy was shown to exist but a third category of 'favourite' cut across both good and bad. To be a favourite of the nurses, the patient did not necessarily have to be good.[36] The effect upon the time and care given to the patient classified as bad has been clearly established. The effect upon the care of the favourite elderly patient has not yet been determined. It could be hypothesised that, in a long-term care institution such as a nursing home, residents are not all treated the same, that in fact favourites will receive more perks and more of the nurse's time and attention. This is something the nurse should be consciously aware of as she discusses with residents their needs and how they can be met.

Most of the care required by aged people who are nearing their death is basically no different from that required by any elderly person. Their nutritional requirements still need to be met, though obviously these will not be the same (see Chapter 3). The physical problems which commonly occur in old age may be more numerous and frequent than a year or six months ago (see Chapter 8). However, there are some practical and emotional problems which are likely to become more apparent.

Practical and emotional problems

Many dying elderly people, often as part of the life review process described earlier, become exceedingly concerned about any 'unfinished business' regarding their relationships. They may feel guilty and want to make amends for some unpleasantness long ago. The nurse should facilitate the bringing together of the two parties, ensuring they have privacy.

Though many elderly people profess not to be afraid of death, when their time for dying seems to be getting close a number will admit to certain fears, particularly if the nurse is a good and sensitive listener. It is common for the dying elderly person not to want to be left alone, especially at night. Consideration should be given by the nurse to ensuring that someone, a relative, friend or nurse, is close by as much as possible. The presence of a night-light might also reduce the person's fear. Another common fear of the dying is that death will be by suffocation, that they will choke to death. A simple explanation of what generally occurs should be given by the nurse. Eleanor Roosevelt expressed a fear when she was dying that she would wake up in the coffin covered by soil. Again, a simple explanation about the certification of death procedure should reassure the person that such a thing just could not occur.

For many elderly people, approaching death brings with it an earnest, sometimes frantic, search for the meaning of life and death. This is more likely to be so in those who have either earlier rejected religion or have never had any. The nurse, however, should ensure that no attempt is made to bring religion to the dying person unless he personally requests it, regardless of relatives' wishes.[37]

The elderly person who is dying may quite suddenly be brought to the realisation that he is leaving the world without leaving behind anything concrete about himself. As a legacy he might like to tape his memoirs, arrange for particular objects of significance to him to be given to his children or grandchildren, or establish a scholarship in his memory.[38] There may be times when the person decides that he wants to make or change his will. The nurse may have to arrange for an appropriate person to come to fulfil the request.

It is evident that the nurse's role in caring for the dying elderly person is quite diverse. However, the nursing staff is not responsible for or able to meet all the dying aged person's needs. Other members of the health care team have various roles and expertise relevant to the care of the dying aged – the occupational therapist, physiotherapist, music therapist, nutritionist, doctor, social worker and clergy – regardless of whether the person is dying at home, in hospital, nursing home or hospice. Nurses, however, are the carers who spend most time with the dying elderly, particularly when they are in nursing homes and the like. They are therefore in a better position to determine the old people's needs and co-ordinate their care.

Conclusion

As members of the health care team, nurses have a sanctioned role to care for bereaved and dying elderly people. But this does not give them *carte blanche* to do as they please. Rather, the nursing interventions planned for each person are made in consultation with that person and modified in response to any change in his/her needs.

Finally, it is essential that nurses maintain their 'TLC' (tender loving care) approach to the dying aged. They also have a responsibility to themselves not to allow the challenge of aiming to give the highest standard of care to these people to overwhelm them. Just as nurses who comfort the bereaved need their own support systems, so too do those caring for the dying.[39] It is therefore their duty to pressure for the establishment of appropriate supports and time, in order to use them for the benefit both of themselves and those for whom they care.

Questions

1. What are the qualities and skills required by the nurse caring for bereaved and for dying elderly people?
2. List the factors which influence elderly people's reactions to a significant loss.
3. What variables should the nurse take into consideration when developing a care plan for bereaved and for dying elderly people?
4. Why should a grieving person be neither sedated nor discouraged from expressing emotion?
5. Discuss the advantages and disadvantages of a bereaved person forming new relationships.
6. What are the reasons for an elderly person's acceptance of death?
7. Is it a pathological response for the grieving person to live as if the deceased were still alive?
8. How should the nurse respond to a bereaved or a dying person who says he/she wants to die?
9. List the principles underlying the care of the bereaved and the dying elderly person.
10. What educational preparation do nurses require to enable them to care for the person who has experienced loss, or who is dying?

References

1. Murray R, Huelskoetter MM, O'Driscoll D. The nursing process in later maturity. New Jersey: Prentice-Hall, 1980.
2. Engel G. Psychological development in health and disease. Philadelphia: W.B. Saunders, 1962.
3. Kastenbaum R. Death, society and human experience. 2nd ed. St Louis: C.V. Mosby, 1981.
4. Schwartz AN, Snyder CL, Peterson JA. Ageing and life: an introduction to gerontology. New York: Holt, Rhinehart and Winston, 1984.
5. Raphael B. The anatomy of bereavement. London: Hutchinson, 1984.
6. Dangott LR, Kalish RA. A time to enjoy the pleasures of ageing. New Jersey: Prentice-Hall, 1979.
7. Swenson WM. Attitudes towards death among the aged. In Feifel H, ed. Death and identity. New York: John Wiley and Sons, 1965.
8. Kalish RA. Death and dying in a social context. In Binstock R, Shanas E, eds. Handbook of ageing and the social sciences. New York: Van Nostrand Reinhold, 1976.
9. Peak DT. The elderly who face dying and death. In Barton D, ed. Dying and death: a clinical guide for caregivers. Baltimore: Williams and Wilkins, 1977.
10. Botwinick J. Ageing and behaviour. New York: Springer Publishing Co. 1973.
11. Butler RN, Lewis MI. Ageing and mental health. St Louis: C.V. Mosby, 1973.
12. Renzenbrink I. Loss and grief in old age. 'Window on progress'. Proceedings of the Third National Conference of the National Association for Loss and Grief, Sydney, 1983.
13. George LK, Weiler SJ. Sexuality in middle and later life. Archives of General Psychiatry 1981; 38: 919-923.
14. Sadock BJ, Kaplan HI, Freedman J, eds. Frigidity, dyspareunia and vaginismus. In Marmor J, ed. The sexual experience. Baltimore: Williams and Wilkins, 1976.
15. Hall A, Selby J, Vanclay F. Sexual ageism. Australian Journal on Ageing 1982; 1: 29-34.
16. Wharton G. Sexuality and ageing. New Jersey: Scarecrow, 1981.
17. Job E. Eighty plus: outgrowing the myths of old age. Queensland: University of Queensland Press, 1984.
18. Thompson LW, Breckenridge JN, Gallagher D, Peterson J. Effects of bereavement on self-perception of physical health in elderly widows and widowers. Journal of Gerontology 1984; 39: 309-314.
19. Dimond M. Bereavement and the elderly: a critical review with implications for nursing practice and research. Journal of Advanced Nursing 1981; 6: 461-470.
20. Smitherman C. Nursing actions for health promotion. Philadelphia: F.A. Davis, 1981.
21. Kimmel DC. Adulthood and ageing. New York: John Wiley and Sons, 1974.
22. Rowles GD. Prisoners of space? Colorado: Westview Press, 1978.
23. Elwell F, Maltbie-Crannell AD. The impact of role loss upon coping resources and life and satisfaction of the elderly. Journal of Gerontology 1981; 36: 223-232.
24. Parkes CM. Bereavement. Harmondsworth: Penguin Books, 1975.
25. Koff TH. Dying, death and survivorship. In Ganikos ML, ed. Counselling the aged. Virginia: American Personnel and Guidance Association, 1979.
26. Brock AM. From wife to widow. Journal of Gerontological Nursing 1984; 10: 8-15.
27. Utley QE, Rasie S. Coping with loss. Journal of Gerontological Nursing 1984; 10: 8-14.
28. Lund DA, Johnson R, Baraki HN, Dimond MF. Can pets help the bereaved? Journal of Gerontological Nursing, 1984; 10: 8-12.

29. Hirst SP, Metcalf BJ. Promoting self-esteem. Journal of Gerontological Nursing 1984; 10:72-77.
30. Eddy JM, Alles WF. Death education. St Louis: C.V. Mosby, 1983.
31. Keith PM. Life changes and perceptions of life and death among older men and women. Journal of Gerontology 1979; 34: 870-878.
32. Pruner M. To the good long life. Great Britain: Macmillan Press, 1978.
33. Jeffers FC, Verwoerdt A. How the old face death. In Busse EW, Pfeiffer E, eds. Behaviour and adaptation in late life. 2nd ed. Boston: Little, Brown and Co, 1977.
34. Yurick AG, Robb SS, Spier BE. The aged person and the nursing process. Connecticut: Appleton-Century-Crofts, 1980.
35. Butler RN. The life review: an interpretation of reminiscence in the aged. In Kastenbaum R, ed. New thoughts on old age. New York: Springer Publishing Co. 1964.
36. Gilliland N, Brunton A. Nurses' typification of nursing home patients. Ageing and Society 1984; 4: 45-67.
37. Carlson D, Wiseman G. Hospice concepts applied to the ageing. In Copp LA, ed. Recent advances in care of the ageing. Edinburgh: Churchill Livingstone, 1981.
38. Ebersole P, Hess P. Toward healthy ageing. St Louis: C.V. Mosby, 1981.
39. Hamric AB. Deterrents to therapeutic care of the dying person — a nurse's perspective. In Barton D, ed. Dying and death: a clinical guide for caregivers. Baltimore: Williams and Wilkins, 1977.

Further reading

Barton D. Approaches to the clinical care of the dying person. In Barton D, ed. Dying and death: a clinical guide for caregivers. Baltimore: Williams and Wilkins, 1977.

Byers JP. Sexuality and the elderly. Geriatric Nursing 1983; 4: 293-297.

Gallagher DE, Breckenridge JN, Thompson LW, Peterson JA. Effects of bereavement on indicators of mental health in elderly widows and widowers. Journal of Gerontology 1983; 38: 565-571.

Kastenbaum RA. Death and bereaved in later life. In Kutscher A, ed. Death and bereavement. Illinois: Thomas, 1969.

Lamerton R. Care of the dying. Harmondsworth: Penguin Books, 1973.

O'Neill S. The nurse and the elderly patient. In Kastenbaum R, ed. New thoughts on old age. New York: Springer Publishing Co. 1964.

Subject Index